CANCER

CANCER

ROBERT M. McALLISTER, M.D.

SYLVIA TEICH HOROWITZ, PH.D.

RAYMOND V. GILDEN, PH.D.

BasicBooks
A Division of HarperCollins*Publishers*

Designed by Ellen Levine

Library of Congress Cataloging-in-Publication Data
McAllister, Robert M., 1922–
    Cancer/Robert McAllister, Sylvia Teich Horowitz, Raymond V. Gilden.
      p. cm.
    Includes bibliographical references and index.
    ISBN 0–465–00845–3 (cloth)
    ISBN 0–465–00846–1 (paper)
      1. Cancer   2. Cancer—Research. I. Horowitz, Sylvia Teich, 1922– .
II. Gilden, Raymond V., 1935– . III. Title.
RC261.M33   1993
616.99'4—dc20   92–53244
                                                   CIP

94 95 96 97 CC/HC 9 8 7 6 5 4 3 2 1

To our devoted families, especially Dodee, Bob, and Joanne, whose forbearance and encouragement made it possible for us to write the book; and to Dr. Robert Huebner, whose energetic quest for the origins of cancer stimulated and supported our efforts and initiated a lifelong friendship between Raymond V. Gilden and Robert M. McAllister.

CONTENTS

PART I
TWENTY YEARS OF CANCER RESEARCH

PART II
THE CANCER PATIENT

PART III
THE TEN MOST COMMON CANCERS

FOREWORD

Cancer is the number-one personal health concern of Americans. Although a million Americans contract the disease every year, many are in the dark about the strides that have been made since millions of dollars became available for cancer research after the passage of the National Cancer Act in 1971.

This book describes the remarkable advances in our understanding of cancer that have taken place in just over twenty years. Most significant to the authors are those that have brought us an increasingly clear picture of the genetic changes that occur as a normal cell becomes transformed into a cancer cell. Most of these genetic changes affect two particular families of genes, protooncogenes and tumor-suppressor genes. Alterations in these genes allow cells to grow in an uncontrolled manner and eventually to metastasize. These genetic changes become, then, a common pathway in the development of cancer. The stimulus to cell replication that creates the potential for errors in the replication of DNA may come from a variety of sources, such as tobacco, saturated fat, or hormones. But the sequence and type of specific genetic changes that occur in cells have much in common.

Some of these genetic changes may be inherited. Most, however, are acquired and thus amenable to therapeutic approaches aimed at restoring the normal state of the cell, free of defective genes. This new field of treatment, called gene therapy, is the most exciting area of current research in cancer treatment.

Much of the progress in cancer research is known only to those engaged in cancer research. Even the practicing physician has difficulty keeping up with the rapid advances in cancer research and with their implications for new methods of diagnosis and treatment. This book attempts to bring together the vast body of information about cancer research over the past two decades into an understandable and readable format. In making sense of this new and exciting research, the authors have done all of us—those in the research community; physicians, nurses, and public health officials directly involved in the delivery of health care; and cancer patients and their families—an important service.

For readers seeking information on currently available diagnosis and treatment regimens, the book has up-to-date information on the various new diagnostic tests, as well as an excellent compilation of information, difficult to find elsewhere, on those factors patients and their families ought to consider in deciding whether to participate in a clinical trial. The book contains all sorts of critical information about who is most likely to develop certain types of cancer, what the relationship between diet and cancer is, what hereditary factors may lead to cancer, plus an invaluable review of the ten most common cancers. Much of this information comes from the protocols of the National Cancer Institute, the largest and most prestigious government-funded research center in the world.

Many cancer patients and their families want to understand the very process of cancer itself, and this book will also meet their needs. Their questions often go unanswered in cancer books meant for the general public, but this book is a rare resource for the reader interested in this technical information, synthesized but not simplified for the lay public. Here interested readers will find answers to many of the questions that they cannot expect their doctors to sit down and explain to them: Is cancer one disease or many? Are cancers caused by viruses or by damage to our genes? What are the tumor-suppressor genes and oncogenes now being mentioned in the lay press as "cancer genes"?

In clear, easy-to-understand language, the authors have assembled a wealth of invaluable information about what we know about the biology of cancer, including the processes of cancer formation. They trace what happens from the moment a single human cell becomes sufficiently damaged to turn cancerous, and why this process often requires many alterations to the cell, taking place over many years. They then follow a cancer cell as it multiplies and metastasizes, leading to full-blown cancers.

No one can now claim that we know all we need to know about cancers, or even that we are close to announcing a cure for cancer. But no one who has studied this research doubts that new diagnostic tools, new treatments, and, perhaps soon, new cures will continue to come about. In the meantime there is great interest in this exciting scientific work, much of it funded with federal money. This book makes it possible for the general public to add to its knowledge and understanding in this important area.

Brian E. Henderson, M.D.
President, The Salk Institute

ACKNOWLEDGMENTS

We have tried to present a balanced, well-informed account of the many facets of cancer. What we report here is the result of the work of legions of scientists, most of whom it would be impossible to acknowledge. Occasional mention of names at least reminds us that there are people behind the advances, examples of the many who spent their careers studying certain aspects of cancer.

We also wish to express our gratitude to colleagues who kindly reviewed early drafts of the book: Sir Michael Stoker, Renato Dulbecco, Peter Vogt, Murray Gardner, Robert Miller, George Donnell, and John Gwinn.

We also acknowledge our dedicated executive secretary, Jeanne Rathbun, not only for her unfailing and cheerful help in the many successive versions of the book that needed to be typed but also for her many critical and useful suggestions.

Finally, it is with deep gratitude that we acknowledge Susan Rabiner, senior editor of Basic Books, for her enthusiastic acceptance and many important directions for the final version of this book, and Linda Carbone, developmental editor of Basic Books, for her skillful editing and gracious interactions with us.

PART I

TWENTY YEARS OF CANCER RESEARCH

Introduction

IN 1971, IN AN EXPRESSION OF UNLIMITED BELIEF IN THE POWER OF well-funded science to conquer disease, President Richard M. Nixon signed into law the National Cancer Act. With it, a "war on cancer" was declared. Funding for cancer research was made a national priority, and the budget of the National Cancer Institute, the cancer-research arm of the National Institutes of Health, the premier government-funded biomedical institute in the world, was increased to an all-time high.

If declaring war on a disease now seems like a dramatic approach—especially in light of the comparatively sluggish response to the AIDS crisis—the statistics on cancer seemed to demand it at the time. And, just two years earlier, the United States had landed a man on the moon; there was a heady sense that cancer, too, could be conquered. Viruses had been implicated in a number of animal cancers, and support seemed to be coalescing within the biomedical research community for the idea that viruses caused some—perhaps many—human cancers as well. The war on cancer was launched in the can-do attitude typical of the times and with the wholehearted support of the nation and the cancer research community.

A glance at more current statistics shows that the war is far from won. Cancer ranks second only to heart disease among causes of death in the United States, accounting for some 23 percent of deaths, or 477,000 per year. There has also been a shift in the kinds of cancer most prevalent in the United States. Between 1973 and 1987, lung cancer increased by 32 percent, melanoma by 83 percent, and non-Hodgkin's lymphoma by 51 percent; there have also been increases in the rates of kidney, brain, prostate, and breast cancers. In 1986, lung cancer surpassed breast cancer as the leading cause of death for women. In spite of advances in chemotherapy, radiation techniques, and surgery, mortality rates from lung cancer, melanoma, multiple myeloma, and non-Hodgkin's lymphoma continued to increase; but those were accompanied by significant decreases in both incidence and mortality for other types of cancer—namely, stomach, cervical, endometrial, testicular, rectal, and Hodgkin's disease. These opposing trends have resulted in a small overall increase in cancer mortality rates (6 percent) over the past forty years. Nevertheless, as the number of deaths from heart disease continues to decrease, those from cancer assume an ever more significant place in the hierarchy of dread diseases. One estimate projects that by the year 2000, cancer may be the leading cause of death in this country. (Preceding statistics are from Henderson et al. 1991, p. 1,131.) A recent Gallup poll commissioned by the American Cancer Society (in Sandroff 1992, p. 18) found that more than half of Americans (59 percent) believe that they are likely to get cancer (compared with 3 percent who expect to get AIDS).

What has happened in cancer research since that infusion of money and effort over twenty years ago? Was it learned that most cancers are caused by viruses? That any are? Do we know what other factors play a significant role in the multistage process that changes healthy cells into cancerous ones? Do we understand metastasis? Do we have any new diagnostic tools or cures to show for all these years of well-funded research?

In late 1991, these questions were asked of Bernadine Healy, the newly appointed director of the National Institutes of Health (NIH) by a congressional committee charged with overseeing government-sponsored medical research. At that point, the government had spent approximately $22 billion on cancer research, and the committee wanted to know exactly what this money had bought—and, implicitly, whether the high level of funding should continue.

Healy gave a spirited response to a somewhat skeptical group of congressmen, noting that scientists had learned a great deal about the causes of cancer at the level of the single cell. She emphasized that "superb basic research" on breast cancer resulted from NIH-funded programs, and that "the most exciting drug to come along in the last fifteen years," taxol, extracted from the Pacific yew tree, was under investigation in the treatment of ovarian cancer (quoted in E. Marshall 1991, p. 1,720).

While it is clear that science still has a long way to go, Healy was accurate in her optimistic assessment of what had already been learned, particularly in regard to breakthroughs in our understanding of the causes and mechanisms of cancer at the level of the single cell. She was also right in pointing out that this new understanding now enables scientists to take original approaches to the treatment of the disease, approaches that may soon yield effective new methods of diagnosing and treating cancer.

Only when such progress is reflected in lower mortality rates will the value of the basic research be apparent to the general public. Hundreds of scientists have contributed their talents to cancer research over the past twenty years; indeed, many of them are our personal friends or former laboratory colleagues. In the interests of clarity and brevity, however, we mention in the text just a handful of the most outstanding researchers.

Because we have been actively engaged in research in the fields of virology and oncology for some thirty years, we have personally felt the excitement that comes from seeing research in this field culminate in an integrated picture of cancer. And in speaking about cutting-edge cancer research before a variety of groups—practicing physicians, nurses, and other health-care professionals, as well as students and diverse segments of the general public—we have discovered that there are many other people as fascinated as we are about how each new piece of the cancer puzzle contributes to a more coherent picture of the disease. Repeatedly, such audiences have asked us to recommend a book, one that is nontechnical and does not talk down to the reader, yet explains what we now understand the cancer process to be. This book is our attempt to fill that need.

In many ways it turned out to be an ambitious undertaking, as we have tried to simplify and correlate vast amounts of research while presenting an accurate picture of the latest advances in cancer research. We also hope to give the reader a sense of the excitement that comes from scientific pursuits and accomplishments. Because our goal is to provide a reader-friendly guide, we have been careful to define all technical and scientific terms and have included a glossary of those terms for easy reference.

Chapter 1 presents a brief history of what was known about cancer prior to 1971. The elucidation in 1953 of the structure of DNA, the genetic material, by James Watson and Francis Crick set off a frenzy of research activity, resulting in our understanding of the normal function and role of DNA as well as the distortions in metabolism that occur when mutations or changes in its structure take place. This phase of scientific endeavor was one of the most intense and exciting in the history of biology and gave rise to the discipline of molecular biology. With the subsequent development of laboratory techniques, research into cancer-causing genetic aberrations could now be studied at the level of the single cell. To understand this research, the reader must know a little about the structure and workings of a normal cell. Chapter 1 includes a simple guide to this basic cell biology.

Chapter 2 tells what happened to the enthusiasm of scientists for the theory that viruses were a main cause of many human cancers. It moves on to the story of how scientific work with one particular family of viruses, the human retroviruses, led to two important breakthroughs. First we relate the story of the discovery of the retrovirus and its mode of reproducing itself in defiance of one of the central dogmas of molecular biology. Then we show how retroviruses were linked to two rare forms of human cancer and ultimately to the deadly disease AIDS. Study of the retrovirus serendipitously led to the discovery of the oncogene, or the first human cancer gene. Once it was learned that retroviruses do not simply infect a cell but often "pick up" a stretch of the cell's own DNA, incorporate it into their own viral genetic material, reproduce, and subsequently infect other cells, we had a scenario that suggested how retroviruses could be linked to the formation of oncogenes.

Chapter 3 provides a historical overview of the discovery of a family of some sixty oncogenes. What has emerged from this impressive research is a realization that such genes are not present in our DNA simply to cause cancer; in developing organisms, from the simple yeast to humans, they play a critical role in stimulating normal cells to multiply. When they function abnormally, they can lead to the unregulated proliferation of cells, a crucial step in the development of cancer.

In chapter 4 we discuss a second class of genes now believed to be related to cancer. Called tumor-suppressor genes, they were discovered in uncommon types of childhood cancers. Interest in this class of gene developed slowly, in the shadow of the great excitement about oncogenes, intensifying only after about a dozen other tumor-suppressor genes were found. One of them was shown to be a factor in more than 50 percent of all cancers in the United States and the United Kingdom.

Chapter 5 presents our understanding of what happens as a normal cell becomes a cancer cell, and as cancer cells migrate to form second, third, or multiple cancerous growths. Perhaps 1 in 100,000 cancer cells acquires the capacity to metastasize, or spread beyond the primary tumor site. These distant tumors are responsible for most deaths from cancer. In this chapter, we describe the process by which metastases form and give the latest information about newly discovered genes that may act to promote or inhibit this process.

Those readers who find these early chapters a bit heavy going may want to skip ahead to parts II and III for now, returning to fill in the biology and research history once they have a feel for the current state of cancer diagnosis and treatment.

Chapter 1

The Human Cell

CANCER IS A DISEASE THAT HAS PLAGUED HUMANS SINCE ANCIENT times. It has been detected in the bones and skulls of Egyptian and Peruvian mummies embalmed as far back as 3000 B.C. Hippocrates, around 400 B.C., first used the term *carcinoma*, from the Greek *karkinoma*, meaning "crab." He likened the disease to a crab because of the clawlike extensions of a spreading cancer. Around A.D. 200 the great Roman physician Clarissmus Galen was the first to refer to fleshy tumors as *sarcomas*, and in 1836, the German pathologist Johannes Müller used the microscope to distinguish between normal and malignant tissues, thus characterizing cancer as a disease of the cell. Cancer cells, when compared to normal cells, were found to be disorganized, abnormal, and inconsistent in size and shape, and they contained misshapen internal structures.

Surprisingly, well into this century cancer was considered by many physicians to be not a single disease but perhaps two hundred different diseases, each with a related but easily distinguishable cause and each calling for its own treatment. It is both sad and sobering to realize that in 1950, when one of us, Robert McAllister, was an intern at a major children's hospital, children newly diagnosed with acute leukemia (cancer of the blood) had a life expectancy of about three months; those with solid tumors (characterized by a lump or mass) had equally dim prognoses.

Four decades later, many forms of cancer can be successfully treated if the primary tumor is surgically removed and has not metastasized, or spread far beyond the original site. Other methods can also lead to a cure in some cases. They include various types of radiation therapy;

TABLE 1.1   *Cancer Survival Trends*

	1960–63 Relative 5-Year Survival Rate (%)		1980–85 Relative 5-Year Survival Rate (%)	
	White	Black	White	Black
All Sites	39	27	51	38
Colon	43	34	55	48
Rectum	38	27	53	39
Breast (females)	63	46	76	64
Uterus, cervix	58	47	67	59
Uterus, corpus	73	31	83	52
Prostate	50	35	73	63

SOURCE: Surveillance and Operations Research Branch, National Cancer Institute, 1990.
NOTE: Epidemiologists keep statistics by race to look for clues to causes.

chemotherapy, which uses compounds that kill cancer cells; photo-therapy, which uses dyes and light waves; and immunotherapy, which enhances immune defenses. Among the newer therapies are those using "biological modifiers" such as interferon, which inhibits cell growth, and interleukin-1, which "arms" certain cells to kill cancer cells, seen as foreign bodies. Interferon and interleukin-1 are protein molecules normally produced in the body by leukocytes. With these treatments, some astonishing cures have been achieved. For instance, Wilms' tumor, a kidney cancer of infants and children, can now be cured in about 90 percent of patients by using a combination of surgery, radiation, and chemotherapy (DeVita et al. 1989, p. 1,624). Other childhood cancers, such as leukemia and tumors of the muscle cells, can sometimes be cured, as can Hodgkin's disease, a lymph-gland cancer found in older children and adults. Despite these examples of remarkable advances in the treatment of certain cancers, however, survival rates of more than five years from the time a patient is diagnosed improved only modestly between the early 1960s and the early 1980s, as table 1.1 shows.

Today scientists see that there is a common pathway for all types of cancer, a view made possible by the startling discovery of two families of genes, the growth-promoting *protooncogenes* and the growth-retarding *tumor-suppressor genes*. A series of alterations in these so-called cancer genes makes possible the uncontrolled growth of a single cell into a life-threatening leukemia or a mass of cancer tissue.

Their unique and crucial role in the origins of cancer suggests entirely new theories about its causes.

Carcinogenesis, or the development *(genesis)* of cancer, is now considered to be a multistep process that begins with a series of specific changes in the DNA of a single cell. The cell and the DNA in the nucleus of the cell are constantly exposed to substances that may alter the genes. These alterations or mutations are almost always repaired by an intricate mechanism with the essential function of preventing havoc in the cell. But if these changes persist in a given cell, that altered cell will breed true—that is, its daughter cells will contain the same altered DNA. In the case of cancer cells, the alteration allows the family of cells derived from a single cell to escape the normal control mechanisms of the cell. Processes related to cell growth and multiplication, such as differentiation, maturation, and proliferation, may then run amok. These unregulated cells will divide rapidly and eventually invade the parent and neighboring tissues to form a tumor. The cancer cells may subsequently dislodge and move to distant sites to establish subcolonies of cancer cells, or *metastases*.

Epidemiologists have concluded that the likelihood of developing cancer increases as an individual ages. This fits the current view of cancer as a slowly progressing disease that involves from two to six or more steps in going from a less malignant to a more malignant and more invasive disease. It also presents the hope that we might learn how to intervene at some point along the way to stop this progression of the disease. (See table 1.2 for a list of the most common forms of cancer.)

Even though scientists may not have had a clear idea until quite recently of what actually causes cancer, there have been extensive scholarly studies on the factors that lead to or are associated with it. A great deal of data was assembled by Sir Richard Doll at Oxford University on environmental factors and chemical carcinogenesis. See tables 1–8 in the appendix for the history of the discovery of these factors: chemicals, radiation, hormones, viruses, heredity, and hazards found in occupational settings and medical procedures. It is now believed that all of these factors may be operating through a common, genetic mechanism—that is, by causing alterations in the DNA of a single cell.

TABLE 1.2 *Common Forms of Cancer*

Cancer	Subtype
Carcinoma	In order of incidence: Skin, Lung, Colon or Rectum, Breast, Prostate, Bladder, Uterus (Endometrium), Oral Cavity and Pharynx, Pancreas, Kidney, Stomach, Ovary, Cervix, Liver, Larynx, Thyroid, Esophagus, Testes
Sarcoma	Soft tissue Bone (osteosarcoma) Cartilage Muscle Uterus
Leukemia	Adult acute lymphocytic leukemia Adult acute myeloid leukemia Childhood acute lymphocytic leukemia Childhood acute myeloid leukemia Chronic lymphocytic leukemia Chronic myelogenous leukemia Hairy-cell leukemia
Lymphoma	Hodgkin's lymphoma Non-Hodgkin's lymphoma
Melanoma	Skin Intraocular
Multiple Myeloma	None
Brain and Nervous Tissue	Spinal cord Astrocytoma Medulloblastoma Ependymoma
Germ Cell Tumors	Seminoma Embryonal Carcinoma Teratocarcinoma Choriocarcinoma Yolk sac tumor
Childhood Cancers	Leukemia Neuroblastoma Wilms' tumor Brain Retinoblastoma

What Is a Tumor?

Although tumors develop frequently as we age, the vast majority of these abnormal cell growths pose little risk to us. The cells of benign tumors, although abnormal, closely resemble adjacent normal cells and may even function like normal cells. The alterations they have sustained in their DNA have not allowed them to escape completely from growth regulation. They remain localized in the tissues where they originated: Benign uterine tumors remain in the uterus; benign liver tumors remain in the liver; benign thyroid tumors remain in the thyroid. Some benign tumors are surrounded by a well-defined capsule of fibrous, scarlike tissue, making it possible to shell the whole thing out surgically. Only rarely do benign tumors become serious medical problems—increasing greatly in size, secreting hormones, or transforming into malignant tumors.

Cancer cells, or malignant tumors, however, are different. When cancers are classified according to the type of cell in which they arise, they fall into three general categories. The first, *carcinomas*, originate in the sheets of cells that cover the skin, respiratory, gastrointestinal, or urinary tracts, or in those lining the various glands, such as breast, prostate, or thyroid. The second category, *sarcomas*, develop in supportive or connective tissues such as bone, fibrous tissue and muscle cells. Both carcinomas and sarcomas are solid tumors. The third category includes *leukemias* and *lymphomas*, which originate in cells that produce circulating white blood cells *(leukocytes)* and in the immune system *(lymphocytes)*. This third group of cancers is usually composed of dispersed cells, although the cells occasionally form solid masses.

Cancer cells can be tentatively identified by microscopic examination. They look different than the normal cells or the benign tumor cells of the tissue in which they are found (see figures 1.1 and 1.2). In general, the more abnormal and bizarre the cells appear, the more malignant the cancer. Although some cancer cells reproduce more rapidly than normal cells—for instance, the cells of certain breast cancers—there are both slow-growing and fast-growing tumors. But cancer cells never stop reproducing, and in time they will outnumber the normal cells around them.

The major characteristic that unambiguously delineates malignant tumor cells from benign cells is that only the former have the ability to invade adjacent tissues and spread to distant sites. In contrast to benign tumors, malignant tumors are not surrounded by a distinct

FIGURE 1.1   Normal Muscle Cell (magnified 18,000 times)

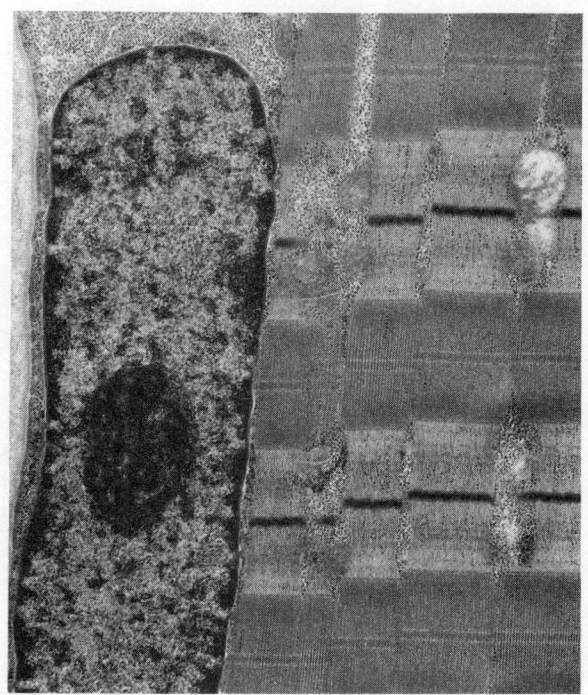

fibrous capsule. Cancer cells may eventually invade the bloodstream and establish colonies far from the original site, a process called *metastasis*. Cells that invade adjacent tissue and metastasize are unquestionably malignant cancer cells.

What Goes On Inside a Cell?

Medical scientists of the past studied disease by observing its effect on the patient as a whole: body temperature, blood pressure, skin coloring, vigor. When the doctor of old asked a patient to stick out his tongue, he was not interested in what was happening in the surface cells of the tongue but in what the appearance of the tongue might tell him about the general condition of the patient. Before the invention of the light microscope by Anton van Leeuwenhoek in the mid-1600s, anatomy consisted of the study of internal organs. This is referred to as gross anatomy because it deals only with structures that can be seen

Figure 1.2   Cancer Cell of Muscle (rhabdomyosarcoma) (magnified 18,000 times)

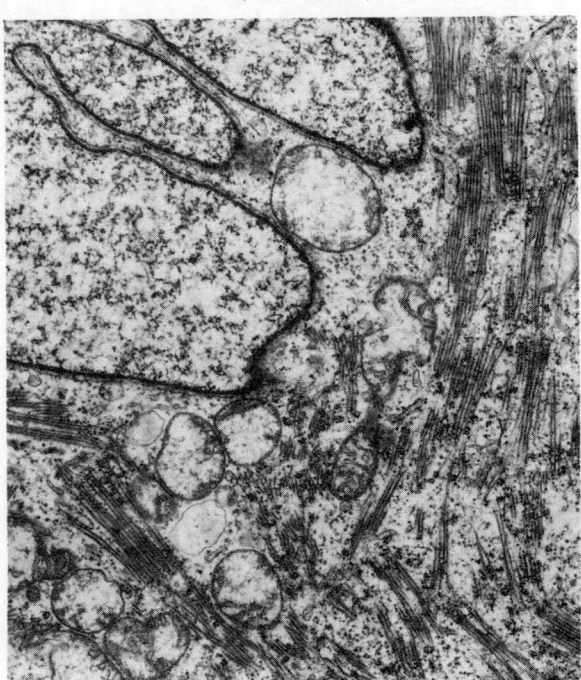

by the naked eye: brain, lung, heart, liver, kidney, and so on. In 1665, Robert Hook observed the honeycomb appearance of a thin slice of cork viewed through a microscope. It reminded him of the cells in a monastery, so the word *cell* came to stand for this most fundamental unit of living things.

Cells of different tissues perform different functions and sometimes even look different: nerve cells resemble long cords and transmit signals from cell to cell; muscle cells resemble large bundles that contract and relax to cause movement; liver cells function as veritable chemical factories. The elegant organization of the human body results from its billions of cells assembled into increasingly complex structures.

Only in the late 1960s with the development of certain laboratory techniques could science move from studying disease *in vivo* (in the living animal) to studying disease *in vitro* (literally, "in glass"—that is, test tubes or glass dishes of cells in nutrient broths). This technique was based on the discovery that certain cells have the remarkable ability to *immortalize*, or continue growing and replicating outside the body provided they are continuously bathed in a nutrient-rich broth. Immortalized cells are important for another reason. Cells that cannot be immortalized can often be kept alive and dividing outside the body if they are grown alongside immortalized cells. Finally, scientists discovered that many types of cells could be kept alive by adding growth factors to their nutrient broths. *Growth factors* are naturally occurring substances in the body whose job, as their name suggests, is to encourage cell growth. To the delight of scientists, these factors also worked when cells were removed from the body and grown in nutrient broths. Armed with these new laboratory techniques, scientists were prepared to launch the study of disease at the level of a single cell.

Cells grow, move, communicate with each other, take in and metabolize food to provide energy, get rid of waste products, and, in most instances, divide or replicate to produce two identical daughter cells. Each cell is separated from its environment by a membrane, which is formed essentially from two layers of fat molecules. At one time this membrane was simply viewed as a barrier that made it possible to keep certain concentration levels of components inside the cell and others outside. Now it is known that embedded in the cell membrane are many proteins that act as gates or receptors, which provide alternative paths into the cell for ions (such as sodium or potassium), foodstuffs (such as glucose or amino acids), and hormones (which are either carried into the cell or set off a chemical response in the membrane itself). Similarly, many growth factors exert their stimulating effect on cell proliferation or division by binding to receptors in the cell membrane. In later chapters we will elaborate on the normal signaling pathways initiated in the membrane of the cell that are subverted in an individual suffering from cancer.

Recent research has revealed that there are also minute channels in cell membranes that allow normal cells to communicate with each other so as to limit their numbers. Any genetic defect resulting in a deficiency of these channels may lead to uncontrolled growth of the cells, a salient characteristic of cancer cells. Can replacement of the defective gene with a normal one reverse the process? That is one approach being explored in cancer research.

Another example of cancer and cell-membrane components comes from studies of breast cancer prognosis. About five years ago it was found that women who had a particular overactive gene in their breast cancer tissue were more likely to suffer a relapse of the disease and more likely to die of it. This gene codes for (that is, leads to the production of) a receptor in the cancer cell membrane. Scientists have very recently been able to pinpoint the breast cancer protein that combines with this receptor and stimulates cancer cell proliferation (Hoffman 1992, p. 1,129). This kind of research and understanding provides clues for designing anticancer drugs that will be able to interfere with the combination of the cancer-produced protein and the membrane receptor and stem the multiplication of cancer cells.

Inside the cell are a variety of subcellular units, smaller specialized structures usually separated by membranes as well. These smaller units are suspended in the *cytoplasm* of the cell, a gel-like fluid that contains many chemical substances required for the cell's metabolism. At one time it was believed that all these units were more or less free-floating in the cytoplasm. But evidence from the high-powered magnification of an electron microscope shows the existence of a delicate lattice that acts as a support for these particles and controls their movement. An exciting consequence of the discovery of this support system is that it tells us that communication among all the cellular components is more direct than previously thought.

Almost every chemical reaction that takes places in living things occurs at a very rapid rate, commensurate with the processes of life. The proteins whose role it is to speed up and control the rates of those reactions are called *enzymes*, the biological catalysts. Later we shall see that the protein products of some protooncogenes act as enzymes for key reactions that control "on/off" switches along the pathways that regulate cell growth and division. If one of these protooncogenes is transformed into an oncogene, it may give rise to a defective enzyme.

What Is DNA?

Now let us turn our attention to the nucleus of the cell, that subcellular body in which the genetic material of the cell resides. Since cancer is a disease involving alterations in genetic material, this site will be the main focus of our discussion of the structure and function of the cell. In the late 1940s the genetic material was determined to be deoxyribonucleic acid, DNA, a large molecule much of whose chemical structure was already known. DNA must possess two extraordinary properties in order to serve as the genetic material: (1) it must be able to direct the making of an exact copy of itself, so that two identical daughter cells can be produced from a parent cell; and (2) it must be able to direct the synthesis of the proper proteins to carry out the functions of living organisms. Although DNA is the material passed from parent to offspring, it is the unique set of proteins that confer the particular characteristics on an individual.

How DNA can perform these fundamental functions became clear in 1953, when James Watson and Francis Crick showed that DNA had the shape not of a long chain, as expected, but of a double helix: two parallel strands coiled around each other and joined by weak linkages that paired together the same two *bases*—the four fundamental units of DNA (adenine pairs with thymine; guanine with cytosine). With this astonishing stroke of insight, Watson and Crick were able to explain how DNA can function as the genetic material. A segment or segments (not necessarily continuous) of the DNA double helix defines a single gene, and these genes are assembled in humans into forty-six chromosomes, called the *human genome*. Human cells contain two copies of each gene, one inherited from each parent—in all some 100,000 genes coding for different proteins and containing approximately three billion base pairs.

This enormous pool is what makes possible each individual's unique set of genes, unique set of proteins, and unique set of characteristics. Only 1 to 2 percent of the pool of base pairs present in all cells is actually expressed as proteins; the remainder is considered nonfunctional ("junk") DNA, and its role is a mystery. Control over whether genes are expressed resides in the *regulator genes*, and just how many are controlled by regulator genes is still unclear. If all the genes were expressed all the time in all the cells, it would lead to chaos. For one thing, it would mean that all the cells would be the same, no specialized liver cells or brain cells or heart cells. Second, all the biochemical reactions, some of which proceed in one direction and some in the reverse direction, would be going on at the same time—a spinning of the biochemical wheels! In addition, it would require a great deal of energy to synthesize all the proteins all the time. The regulator genes therefore play an extremely important role in normal metabolism, and it is now universally accepted that they also have a crucial role in the initiation of cancer.

How Do "Errors" in DNA Relate to Cancer?

As explained, the DNA in humans resides in the nucleus, a relatively sequestered region of the cell that is not subject to as many stresses as the rest of the cell. The message in the DNA must be copied onto another nucleic acid, called RNA, which can travel from the nucleus to the place where proteins can be made. A protein is a large molecule consisting of amino acids linked together in a chain. The RNA, having copied the "code" from the DNA, assembles the required amino acids and directs the synthesis, or "translation," that will incorporate the amino acids into the protein in the specific order or sequence dictated by the arrangement of bases originally found in the DNA for that gene. Any alteration in the bases in the DNA, such as those that occur in the cancer process, may lead to an altered RNA and an error in the amino acids assembled. A different protein will result, which may have a serious effect on cell function.

Alterations in the DNA of cells may occur in many ways. Errors may occur during DNA duplication; one chromosome may drop bits of itself that become attached to another chromosome; environmental factors such as ultraviolet rays from the sun, X rays, or toxins in foods may damage DNA. Most of these genetic errors are repaired, but when they occur at certain sites near regulator genes, the cell's ability to control the "turning on" and "turning off" of important genes may be disrupted. The possibility of cancer initiation then becomes greater.

A specific example of such a gene alteration that has a dramatic effect on skin cells has recently been reported. The incidence of squamous-cell carcinoma (which affects about 100,000 people annually in the United States) was for a long time correlated with excessive exposure to the sun, especially to ultraviolet-B radiation, which penetrates to the inner layers of skin. Now it has been determined that a precise genetic change is caused by this single carcinogenic agent: the change in the DNA of these squamous cancer cells occurs in a tumor-suppressor gene (Vogelstein and Kinzler 1992, p. 210). Thus, when the normal base sequence in that gene is changed as a result of exposure to radiation, the gene is no longer effective in performing its job. Uncontrolled squamous-cell proliferation, or cancer, may result.

Can Cancer Be Inherited?

Now that we have looked briefly at the role of DNA and the idea that carcinogenesis involves a stepwise alteration in certain genes, we can begin to answer some important questions about individual susceptibility to the disease: Does cancer run in families? Is a predisposition to cancer inherited? The answer to both is a qualified yes.

Practically all forms of cancer in humans exhibit a tendency to aggregate or cluster. Are these cancers associated with specific gene alterations? Again, the answer appears to be yes. Several mutations or alterations in one tumor-suppressor gene, the p53 gene, have been shown to be the most common genetic mutations observed in human cancer, found in 70 percent of colon cancers, 30 to 50 percent of breast cancers, 50 percent of lung cancers, and all small-cell lung cancers (one of the two major types of lung cancer; Levine 1992, p. 1,351).

Since an individual inherits one gene from each parent, a parent carrying a defective p53 gene in an egg or a sperm cell can contribute that defective gene to the fertilized egg cell and to every body cell that develops into the embryo and ultimately the offspring. That individual starts with one defective copy of the tumor-suppressor gene, requiring only the loss of function in the second copy to knock out the down-regulation of cell proliferation governed by that gene. As researchers in the field have pointed out, however, the fact that an individual inherits one defective p53 gene does not mean that cancer will develop at an early age or that all the body cells will be equally susceptible to an alteration of the second copy (Levine 1992).

In contrast to the inheritability of mutations in tumor-suppressor genes, mutations in the oncogenes seem to arise spontaneously, in response to the myriad of stresses to which genes are subjected over the lifetime of the individual. No naturally occurring inherited forms of such mutations have yet been demonstrated.

When I. B. Weinstein, a renowned investigator in the field of cancer research, said that in cancer the genome is "shot to hell," he was referring to the current view that as many as ten or more distinct mutations may have to accumulate in critical genes before a cell becomes cancerous. Exploration of the issue of cancer inheritability is being vigorously pursued in workshops under the aegis of the National Cancer Institute and the National Center for Human Genome Research.

With this introduction to the current concept of cancer, the definition of some useful terms for our subsequent discussion, and an overview of basic cell biology, we are ready to describe the important role played by retroviruses in the process of carcinogenesis.

Chapter 2

Retroviruses

R ETROVIRUSES ARE CONSIDERED THE MOST IMPORTANT FAMILY OF viruses, certainly with respect to carcinogenesis. Most retroviruses do not cause disease, but a few do and are also responsible for the majority of cancers in a wide variety of animals. Leukemias and lymphomas in chickens, mice, domestic cats, and cattle, as well as some cancers in monkeys and apes, are caused by retroviruses. Once the connection between retroviruses and animal cancer was established and it was further shown that retroviruses could transform infected cells into cancer cells *in vitro*, it seemed reasonable to postulate that retroviruses would also play a major role in human cancer. But this has not proved to be the case. Despite extensive efforts to isolate retroviruses from every type of human cancer, only two retroviruses have been found to be associated with two forms of human leukemia, diseases that account for only a minuscule proportion of all cancer cases. Retroviruses do, however, cause AIDS.

What Is a Retrovirus?

Viruses are the smallest form of living organism. They consist basically of a central core composed of their genetic material, either RNA or DNA, and some proteins, most of which form the outer coat. Figure 2.1 illustrates retrovirus particles observed by electron microscopy. Because they are such simple organisms, they survive in nature only by infecting other living cells and then using the infected cells' machinery to reproduce themselves. During this process the RNA or

FIGURE 2.1   Electron Micrograph of a Type B Retrovirus, Mouse
Mammary Tumor, Virus-Infected Cell (magnified 75,000 times)

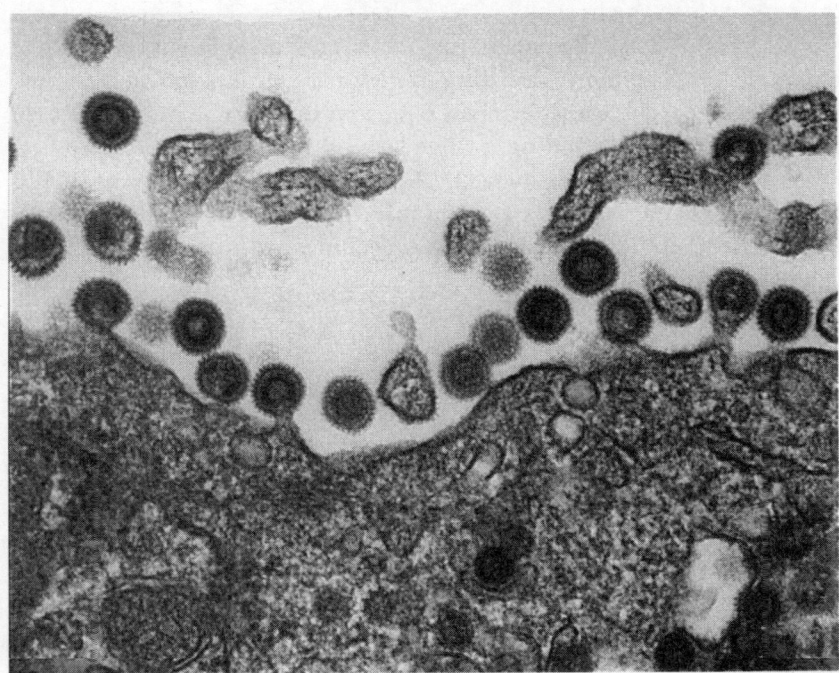

This figure shows a number of particles in various stages of maturation. There are
several particles in the process of budding from the cell surface (attached by stalks),
a number of newly released virus particles with a well-defined circular internal
ring (nucleoid), and several mature particles with the nucleoid located in an
eccentric position within the virus particle (example at far left). This particular
virus, as distinguished from most others in the family, also develops its core
structure within the cytoplasm of the cell. External "spikes," representing the
envelope protein, are also clearly seen on the surface of the virus particle.

DNA is assembled along with the virus coat, following which the
infected host cell is usually killed and releases large numbers of complete new virus particles.

Retroviruses differ from other viruses in their method of replicating.
Following attachment and penetration of the retrovirus particle into
an infected cell, the RNA genome, or genetic information, of the
retrovirus is transcribed into a copy of DNA by a unique enzyme called
reverse transcriptase, which is contained within the virus particle.
The DNA copy is then integrated or inserted into the DNA of the

infected host cell. This incorporated retroviral DNA serves as the template from which new retroviral RNA is copied, and this leads to the synthesis in the host cell of retroviral proteins. These new proteins are translated from the retroviral RNA and assembled around the retroviral RNA genome, resulting in new retroviruses in the host cell. The new retrovirus particles then bud from the surface of the infected cell, usually without killing it. The surviving cell with the retroviral DNA incorporated in its own DNA will constantly release more retroviruses and transmit the genetic information from one cell generation to the next. This retroviral DNA becomes a permanent part of the cell—perhaps, as some evidence suggests, a significant portion of the mammalian genome.

The finding that these viruses contain reverse transcriptase was startling. It contradicted the central dogma of molecular biology, which held that in all organisms DNA is transcribed into RNA which in turn is translated into proteins. The enzyme found in these viruses transcribes RNA into DNA—hence the names *reverse transcription* and *retrovirus.*

The Role of Retroviruses in Carcinogenesis and Gene Therapy

In the 1970s, the first oncogene, or cancer gene, was discovered in combination with the genome of the Rous sarcoma virus of chickens. Apparently the retrovirus has the capacity to "pick up" a gene from the infected animal cell and incorporate it into its own genome. This gene, designated *src,* has been found in the DNA genomes of all organisms from yeast to man. When a gene is so conserved—that is, when it has the same base composition in such a wide range of organisms—it is assumed to be involved in some essential process. *Src* was shown to be involved in the regulation of the growth of cells, a process that is fundamental to the normal development of an organism. The combination of such a normal gene with a retroviral genome can, however, alter the normal gene in a number of ways that may lead to the development of cancer:

1. It can relocate the normal gene to a different site in the chromosomes.
2. It can cause that gene to be overexpressed or amplified, resulting in the production of excessive protein product.

3. It can cause the gene to mutate or undergo a genetic alteration so that it can no longer perform its normal function.

Any of these effects can transform the normal cellular gene—the protooncogene—into an active cancer gene—the oncogene.

As previously mentioned, the milestone scientific discovery of the 1970s was of reverse transcriptase. For this landmark discovery, David Baltimore and Howard Temin shared the Nobel Prize in Medicine and Physiology in 1975 with Renato Dulbecco, who was cited for his contribution to the basic understanding of the interaction between viruses and the genetic material of the cell. Reverse transcriptase has had a profound effect not only on the central dogma describing the transfer of genetic information but on the field of genetic engineering, which uses retroviruses to alter the genotype (genetic constitution) of an animal or human cell. Retroviruses are crucial players in the emerging field of gene therapy because they contain the enzyme reverse transcriptase. It is estimated that there are some four thousand diseases that result from the presence of a defective gene or the absence of the normal gene. Gene therapy is designed to provide the cell with the normal gene.

In the 1980s, Richard Mulligan at the Whitehead Institute in Cambridge, Massachusetts, first used a retrovirus as the vehicle for inserting a normal gene into the DNA of the host cell. Cancer such as non-small-cell carcinoma of the lung is among the diseases targeted for treatment using these new techniques. Other diseases that will be the subject of experimental trials include cystic fibrosis, severe combined immune deficiency (SCID), hemophilia, and familial hypercholesterolemia.

In these trials, cells removed from the patient are induced to divide *in vitro.* The retrovirus used as a vector must have some of its own genes deleted to make certain it can no longer act as an infectious agent or even replicate. This disabled retrovirus is then attached to a normal replacement gene that contains a promoter, which acts to stimulate production of the protein for which the gene codes. The retrovirus and its genetic cargo are then introduced into the deficient cells and incorporated into their cellular DNA. The resultant cells are injected into the patient. The daughter cells derived from this altered cell will all contain the retroviral DNA and the newly inserted gene. In theory (but not yet in practice) this kind of gene therapy could provide a lifetime cure.

The use of retroviruses in gene therapy does entail some risk, even assuming that the retrovirus does not revert to its original genetic form and become an infectious agent. The danger lies in the fact that the retrovirus carrier inserts itself randomly into the cellular DNA and may in this process transform a protooncogene into an oncogene, or inactivate a tumor-suppressor gene and thus initiate cancer. Although investigators believe this risk to be extremely small, safety is still a primary focus.

Another interesting discovery concerning retroviruses and their role in carcinogenesis is their ability to relocate a segment of their DNA to a different site in the chromosome. Some retroviruses have a molecular anatomy that resembles so-called DNA insertion elements, which have been found in maize, bacteria, yeast, and fruit flies. Like these "jumping genes," retroviral DNA can transpose from one site in the DNA to another. Such transpositions are believed to result in the activation of some cellular or host genes or the inactivation of others, steps in the progressive stages leading to cancer. As often happens in science, work that at the time appears to be an anomalous and isolated phenomenon is suddenly brought into the mainstream of scientific progress. The first experiments providing evidence of the existence of transposable regions of DNA in cells came from the experiments on maize plants performed by Barbara McClintock in the 1950s. Her results indicated that some genes do in fact move from one position to another or even to different chromosomes, but this finding remained on the periphery of scientific thought as the revolution in molecular biology unfolded. Not until the 1980s, when new supporting evidence emerged in yeast, bacteria, and Drosophila, has the phenomenon of mobile, transposable genes been seen as a fundamental process. McClintock's contribution was recognized by the awarding of a Nobel Prize in 1983. It has since been shown that some retroviruses can behave in the same way, and their transposition lead to cancer in animals.

Retroviruses and Cancer in Animals

The role of retroviruses in the induction of cancer in animals was elaborated in the 1960s and, as mentioned earlier, spurred the search for a retroviral role in human cancer. Retroviruses have been shown to be associated with the induction of cancer in experimental in vitro systems and, indeed, in some leukemias and sarcomas of animals. The natural history of retrovirus-induced cancer in chickens has changed dramatically since Rous's early studies of sarcomas in that species. None of those cancers was classified as leukemia or lymphoma, and no leukemia retroviruses were detected. With the present-day close crowding of chickens in large-scale commercial breeding facilities, however, there has been a profound increase in the spread of leukemia retroviruses, resulting in a devastating loss of chickens to this disease.

Of particular interest to cat lovers is the incidence of feline leukemia and lymphoma. These diseases are widely disseminated in cat populations, infecting approximately 1 in 1,000 domesticated cats. The retrovirus associated with these diseases is spread horizontally—that is, between kittens or young cats by exchange of virus-containing saliva—but may also be transmitted vertically, from mother to fetus *in utero*, since newborn kittens harboring the retrovirus later develop lymphomas. Although most retrovirus-infected cats fortunately do not develop any disease, a higher-than-normal incidence of leukemia and lymphomas is found in households where many kittens and young cats live together.

The *f*eline *l*eukemia retrovirus (FeLV) appears to be unusually competent in "picking up" oncogenes from its natural host. To date, ten such oncogenes derived from cat cells have been discovered in cat retroviruses. The pet cat is, therefore, an excellent species from which cellular oncogenes can be isolated after they have recombined with FeLV. A number of these oncogenes have been associated with solid tumors of cats.

A worrisome discovery made in a number of laboratories, including our own, is the finding that cat retroviruses can infect and transform human cells into cancer cells *in vitro*. Can cat leukemia and sarcoma retroviruses in fact cause cancer in humans? Extensive studies of human serum, including specimens from veterinarians who are exposed to many cats with these diseases, indicate that feline retroviruses do not infect humans, do not induce an antibody response, and have not been shown to cause any type of cancer in humans (Gardner et al. 1977, p. 1,250).

Leukemia and lymphomas are also the most common cancers occurring in cattle. A considerable increase in the incidence of these diseases has been observed during the past three decades in Germany, Denmark, Sweden, the United States, and other countries. About 40 percent of the cases occurred in herds, more commonly in dairy cows than in beef cattle (Gross 1983, p. 63). The *b*ovine *l*eukemia retrovirus (BLV) that causes the disease can be transmitted vertically, from one generation to another, or horizontally, from infected to noninfected animals. Hence the infected herds show multiple cases of the disease.

Retroviruses and Cancer in Humans

As it became evident that the majority of cancers in a variety of animals—chickens, mice, cats, and cows—are caused by retroviruses, scientists began to focus their attention on the role of retroviruses in human cancer. Extensive efforts were made from the late 1960s through 1979 to detect and isolate human retroviruses from cancer tissue and leukemic blood cells. This wide-ranging search for retroviruses extended from analyses of human cancer tissue, using the high-powered electron microscope, to attempts to detect either retroviral antigens or the antibodies produced in response to these antigens.

All proved futile. Methods that had proved successful in the isolation of retroviruses from a number of animal species failed to detect retroviruses in humans, but they did provide strong evidence against horizontal infection (from one human to another) with any of the known mammalian retroviruses. With recent advances in DNA technology, including more sensitive detection techniques, clear evidence has now been obtained for the presence of noninfectious retroviral sequences in human cells. In fact, it is now estimated that 0.1 to 0.2 percent of the human genomic DNA consists of retroviral DNA. Based on the analysis of their nucleotide sequences, many of these retroviral genes appear to be defective and so the retrovirus does not multiply.

Finally, in 1980, the search for a retrovirus associated with disease in humans was successful. Robert Gallo and his co-workers at the National Cancer Institute described the first bona fide retrovirus associated with an aggressive form of adult leukemia or a lymphoma that originates in T-lymphocytes. This retrovirus, designated *human T-cell leukemia virus* (HTLV-I), was isolated from a patient with adult T-cell leukemia. (T-cells are the type of white blood cells called lymphocytes derived from the thymus gland.) Interestingly, the isolation of HTLV-I resulted from the convergence of two sets of studies in Gallo's laboratory: efforts to culture T-cells, a component of the immune system, and efforts to isolate the retrovirus that causes T-cell leukemia. The investigators were studying a protein growth factor acting on T-cells. When this growth factor, called *interleukin-2* (IL-2), was added to cultures of T-cells, it stimulated one subset of these cells to grow indefinitely, and these became a site for the growth of the retrovirus, HTLV-I, thus facilitating its isolation.

Adult T-cell leukemia is a disease that was first discovered in Kyushu and Shikoku, the southernmost islands of Japan. Patients show symptoms of skin lesions as well as an enlarged liver and spleen and usually survive no longer than three to four months after the onset of these symptoms. The disease occurs in clusters of cases in lower socioeconomic groups in rural areas of southwestern Japan, Africa, the Caribbean islands, and the southeastern United States. The adult T-cell leukemia retrovirus isolated by Japanese scientists, designated ATL, was subsequently shown to be identical to HTLV-I. HTLV-I is transmitted through sexual contact and through transfusion of infected blood. Transmission also occurs from mother to infant by means of breast milk. The interval between virus infection and overt disease varies from a few years to as long as forty years.

Once HTLV-I was isolated, tests were devised to detect antibodies directed against the retroviral proteins that acted as antigens. These tests revealed that about 1 in 1,000 individuals were infected with HTLV-I in certain areas. However, fewer than 1 in 100 individuals who were infected with, and had antibodies to, the retrovirus ever developed the adult T-cell leukemia. In 1982, a retrovirus closely related to HTLV-I, called HTLV-II, was discovered in the United States in a patient with hairy-cell leukemia. Infection with this retrovirus is rare.

The quest for human retroviruses had led only to these two, which are certainly not the cause of the majority of human cancers, until the discovery in 1983–84 of a third: *human immunodeficiency virus*, or HIV, the AIDS virus, which belongs to a different subfamily of retroviruses from HTLV-I and HTLV-II.

How Do Retroviruses Cause Cancer?

How retroviruses cause cancer is best answered by first considering the molecular anatomy of the three classes of retroviruses, shown in figure 2.2. Those retroviruses designated chronic leukemia viruses have only three genes, *gag, pol,* and *env,* and long terminal repeats (LTR) of ribonucleic acids at each end of the genome. A second class of retrovirus, designated the acute leukemia and sarcoma viruses, has acquired a fourth gene, an oncogene, that often partially replaces some of the usual three retroviral genes. The third class of retroviruses, called

FIGURE 2.2 Three Classes of Retrovirus

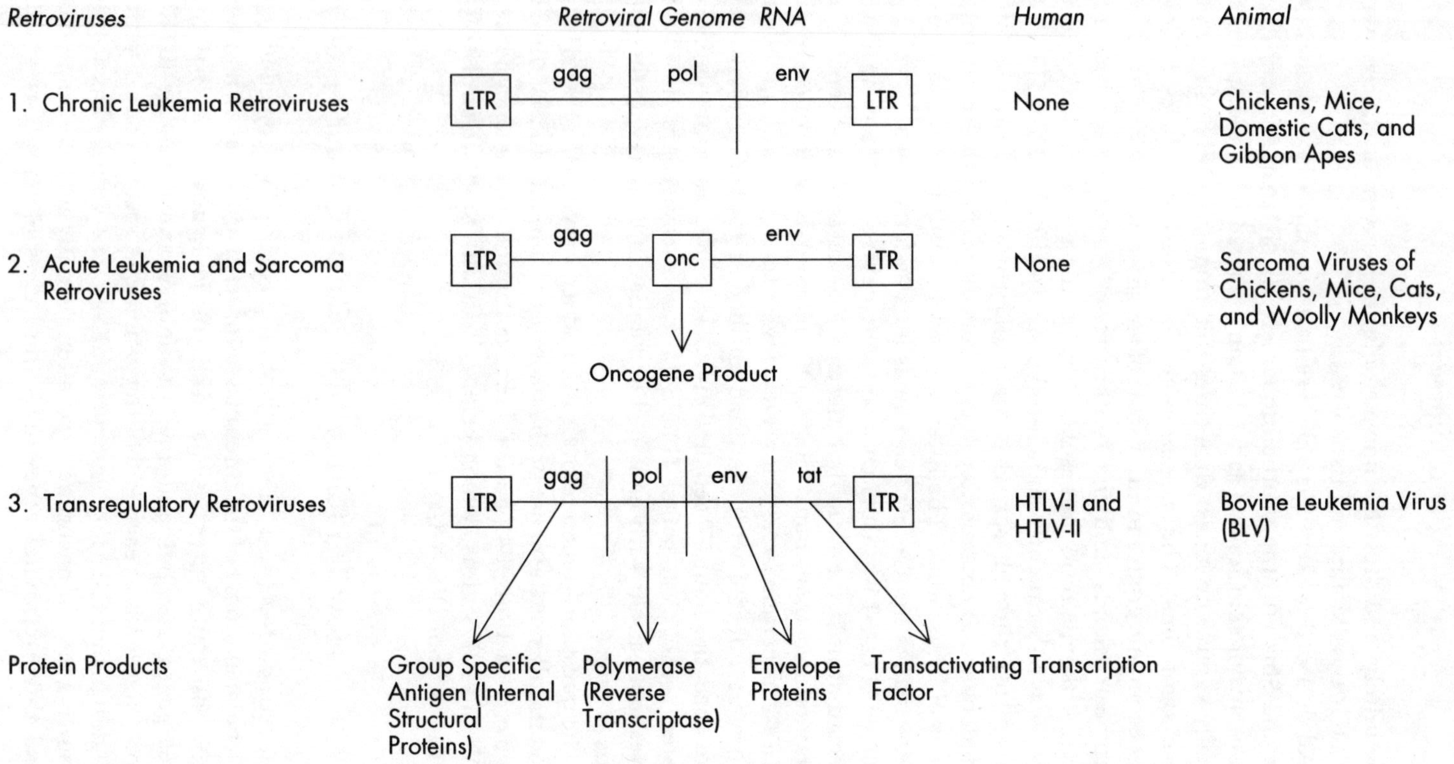

Retroviruses	Retroviral Genome RNA	Human	Animal
1. Chronic Leukemia Retroviruses	LTR — gag — pol — env — LTR	None	Chickens, Mice, Domestic Cats, and Gibbon Apes
2. Acute Leukemia and Sarcoma Retroviruses	LTR — gag — onc — env — LTR → Oncogene Product	None	Sarcoma Viruses of Chickens, Mice, Cats, and Woolly Monkeys
3. Transregulatory Retroviruses	LTR — gag — pol — env — tat — LTR	HTLV-I and HTLV-II	Bovine Leukemia Virus (BLV)

Protein Products

Group Specific Antigen (Internal Structural Proteins)

Polymerase (Reverse Transcriptase)

Envelope Proteins

Transactivating Transcription Factor

LTR = long terminal repeat, insertional element

transregulatory retroviruses, includes HTLV-I and HTLV-II as well as bovine leukemia virus. In addition to the three usual genes, these contain additional genes that are not oncogenes. The protein products of these extra genes may act at a distance to activate other cellular genes.

The chronic leukemia retroviruses that do not have an oncogene cause most of the leukemias seen in chickens, mice, and cats both in nature and in laboratory studies. The leukemias caused by these chronic leukemia retroviruses usually occur in older animals in nature, or after many months if the retroviruses are injected into young animals in the laboratory.

The basis for the leukemia is that the injected chronic leukemia virus, without an oncogene, inserts itself in the chicken cell DNA near the c-*myc* protooncogene. Here the viral LTR (see figure 2.2) causes overexpression of the c-*myc* gene. Such overexpression of a protooncogene protein product may lead to cancer because these proteins act at critical steps in growth factor signaling pathways that control cell proliferation or multiplication as well as other basic differentiation patterns in the cell.

By contrast, the acute leukemia or sarcoma retroviruses, such as the Rous sarcoma virus or the mouse, cat, and woolly monkey sarcoma viruses, have actually acquired a cellular oncogene as part of the retroviral DNA. When these retroviruses are injected into appropriate hosts they cause an acute disease, usually a sarcoma, soon after the infection. Similarly, when they infect cultured cells *in vitro*, something like microtumors are visible in the culture after a few hours.

A third mechanism seems to operate in the case of the transregulatory retroviruses. These retroviruses, which include the human HTLV-I, HTLV-II, and the related bovine leukemia virus, have three novel genes in their RNA genome but do not contain an oncogene. One of these, the *tat* gene, codes for a protein that activates retroviral (LTR) genes at distant sites. This activation increases the rate of transcription of the retroviral genes that lead to the leukemia (The name *tat* stands for transactivator of transcription.) Besides activating transcription of the retroviral genes, *tat* can also act at a distance and cause transcription of cellular, nonviral genes, including the interleukin-2 (IL-2) gene associated with T-cell proliferation. Thus, the mechanism by which HTLV-I causes adult T-cell leukemia, although not completely clear at present, could include activation of IL-2 gene and immortalization or uncontrolled continuing proliferation of

T-cells. Such a mechanism would account for the large numbers of T-cells in patients with this form of leukemia.

Following infection of animals with HTLV-I, a DNA copy of the retrovirus RNA gene is integrated into the cellular DNA of the leukemia T-cells. Although the retroviral DNA is integrated into the DNA of the leukemic T-cells at different sites in different patients, in a given individual patient the retroviral DNA is integrated into the same location in all the leukemic T-cells. This indicates that the leukemia in that patient was derived from a single infected cell. The HTLV-I leukemia is therefore a family of cells derived from a single cell. Similarly, in bovine T-cell leukemia, the DNA of BLV integrates into bovine cellular DNA at a different site in the leukemic cells of each infected animal but in the same site in the leukemia cells of a given infected animal.

We have discussed three proposed molecular mechanisms describing how retroviruses can cause cancer in humans and animals. Our focus now moves to the role of retroviruses as activators of protooncogenes, transforming them into oncogenes.

Chapter 3

Oncogenes

Since their discovery in the 1960s, oncogenes have become one of the most thoroughly investigated classes of genes. In fact, scientists in the field declared 1982 the "year of the oncogene." That same year Michael Bishop, a future Nobel Laureate, succinctly described why there was so much excitement about oncogenes: "They are genes that cause cancer. They were first found in viruses, but their evolutionary history implies that normal vertebrate cells have genes whose abnormal expression can lead to cancerous growth" (Bishop 1982). The cascade of information about oncogenes that began flowing out of research laboratories in the 1960s continues unabated today.

What Is an Oncogene?

Are oncogenes, as their name implies (*onc* is from the Greek word for "tumor"), the genes that cause cancer? Or are they actually genes involved in normal growth and differentiation that only inadvertently cause cancer? The answer to both questions appears to be yes. Indeed, one of the most revealing discoveries of the current research on the causes of cancer is that in each cell in our bodies, there are a large number of genes, perhaps three hundred to four hundred, whose normal function is to control critical cellular functions. These normal genes, or protooncogenes, can be subverted, or altered, in a variety of ways that may turn them into oncogenes. Close to sixty such oncogenes have already been shown to be involved in carcinogenesis, both naturally occurring and experimentally induced.

The protooncogenes are the targets of a wide range of environmental insults, ranging from chemical (such as foods, drugs, and, equally important, products of normal cell metabolism) to physical (such as X rays and ultraviolet light) to biological (such as errors in DNA replication). If the protooncogene is altered or mutated as a result of these insults and is not repaired by the intricate processes in place in the cell, the resulting oncogene may no longer be able to code for the proper protein product to perform the normal cell function.

Since oncogenes were discovered as part of retroviruses that cause cancer, they were aptly named "cancer genes." By the time it was discovered that oncogenes are, in fact, mutated forms of normal genes that are involved in a variety of vital cell functions, it was too late to revise the literature and rename the genes. Developmental biologists are less than delighted with this terminology, implying as it does that the major role of protooncogenes is to give rise to oncogenes—an inaccurate description.

The Discovery of Oncogenes

Direct attempts to isolate "cancer genes" from the genome of humans or other vertebrates would entail locating and separating out some sixty genes from the tens of thousands of genes in the chromosomes—a monumental, well-nigh impossible task. Fortunately, the retrovirus does the job for us, by incorporating the host oncogene into its own genome. Retroviruses have, in fact, acted with great precision as vehicles for the isolation of most of the known oncogenes in a wide variety of vertebrates—but not in humans. Oncogenes in humans have been identified by other techniques, though in many cases requiring the information gained from the structures of the oncogenes isolated from retroviruses.

The story of the retroviruses as carriers of oncogenes begins around 1911 with the discovery that the Rous sarcoma virus (RSV) is responsible for solid tumors (sarcomas) in chickens. Some sixty years later, in 1970, Peter Duesberg and Peter Vogt, working independently, observed that the genome of the transforming RNA tumor virus, RSV, is larger than the genome of nontransforming retroviruses. When it became possible to identify the genes of the two types of retroviruses, it was learned that the genomes of the retroviruses that cause the transformation contain an additional gene, an oncogene named *src.*

In 1976 came the highly significant finding that the same *src* oncogene was a part of the human genome, but not incorporated into a retroviral genome. Indeed, scientists were able to demonstrate that a single *src* gene, or a few copies of it, was "conserved" in the DNA in the whole spectrum of organisms from yeast to humans. When a gene is so conserved—that is, when it remains largely intact—in such a wide range of diverse species, it is a good indication that this gene plays some critical role in cell function. In this case, that critical role is cellular growth and development.

Table 9 in the appendix lists the human oncogenes isolated from a variety of cancers, along with their chromosome location, where known. The curious three-letter abbreviations used to designate an oncogene or a protooncogene are readily understandable only to experts in the field. The oncogenes found within a retroviral genome have been designated v-*onc;* their counterparts detected in the chromosomal DNA of all species as cellular oncogenes are c-*onc,* or protooncogenes. Since no human oncogenes have been found to be associated with a retroviral genome, all the human oncogenes are mutated c-*onc* genes.

The anatomy of oncogenes is typical of that of other known genes. They are constructed of a linear array of the four base pairs that constitute the double-stranded DNA molecules. Some differences have been detected between the *onc* genes present in the viruses (v-*onc*) and those in cells (c-*onc*). These differences have mainly consisted of the loss of some base pairs in the v-*onc* that apparently were excised when the virus incorporated the c-*onc* into its genome. Because of the current explosion of new techniques available to the molecular biologist, it has been possible to obtain the exact sequence of DNA base pairs in a number of oncogenes.

How Are Oncogenes Detected?

We have already explained the insertion of oncogenes into retroviruses. These altered retroviruses can induce various types of cancer in animals and can also be detected by transforming cells in culture

into cancer cells. An important technique for detecting human oncogenes was discovered in 1974. Called *transfection*, the original procedure involved the isolation of the DNA from rat tumors that had been
induced by Rous sarcoma virus containing the v-*src* gene, spreading
this DNA on the culture of normal chicken cells, and observing the
formation of colonies of transformed cells. The oncogene in the rat
tumor cell moved ("transfected") into the normal chicken cells and
was responsible for their transformation into cancer cells. Reasoning
by analogy, many researchers believed it might be possible to detect
transforming genes in DNA isolated from human tumors by transfecting them into normal cells and producing colonies of transformed
cells.

The experiments of Robert Weinberg at the Massachusetts Institute
of Technology were notably successful. He tested DNA from human
tumors for its capacity to transform mouse cells (from the cell line NIH
3T3) into cancer cells. DNA extracted from human tumors of the
bladder, colon, and lung was spread onto cultures of these normal
mouse cells and produced colonies of transformed cells. When these
transformed cells were inoculated into mice, tumors were formed at
the site of inoculation (see figure 3.1). So the technique of transfection
could now be used to detect oncogenes in DNA isolated from human
cancers.

These two experimental techniques, one from the animal transfection experiments and the other from the human studies, converged
dramatically when it was determined that the DNA isolated from
human cancer tissue owed its transfecting activity to oncogenes that
were homologous (similar in composition of bases) to members of
the v-*ras* oncogene family found in retroviruses. The *ras* oncogene
family, as we will discuss, is an important component of the signal-
transduction system leading to cellular proliferation.

With this technique, a number of transfecting oncogenes in addition to the *ras* family have been detected in the DNA isolated from a
variety of human cancers: breast cancer, neuroblastoma, stomach and
colon cancer, Kaposi's sarcoma, and cancer of the bladder, colon, lung,
pancreas, ovary, and skin. Although this mouse cell line has a particular utility in these experiments, overall only about 20 percent of
human cancers yield DNA capable of transforming these cells, indicating that the techniques do have limitations.

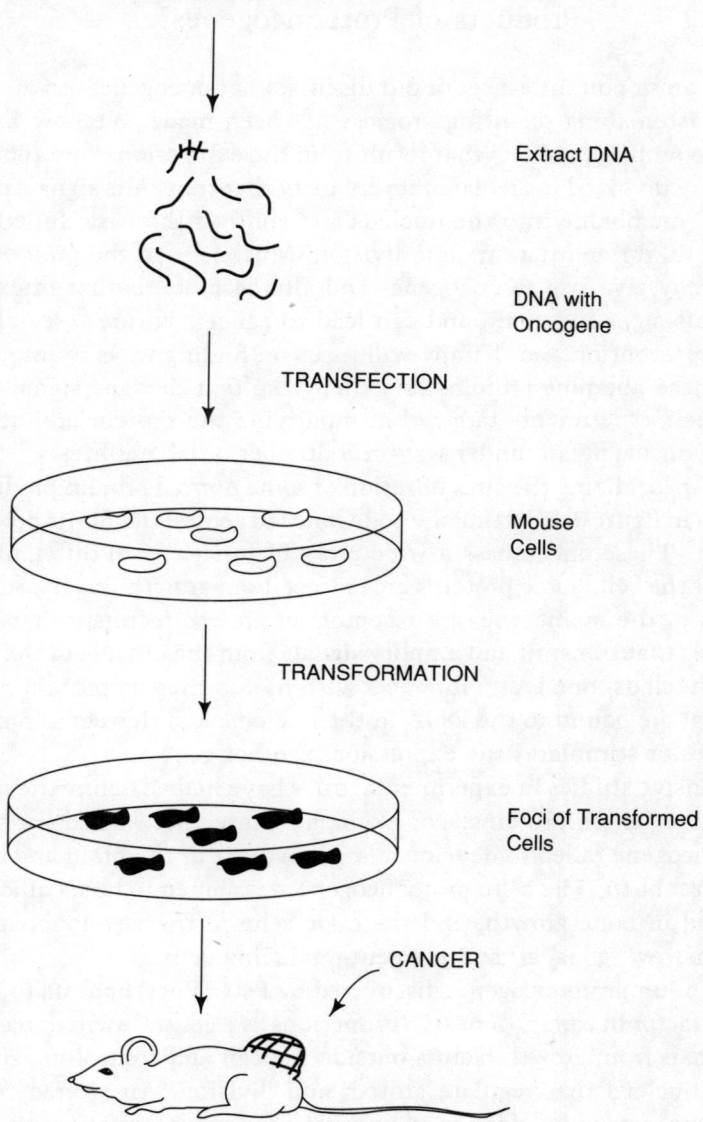

FIGURE 3.1 Oncogene Transfer by Transfection

HUMAN CANCER TISSUE

Extract DNA

DNA with
Oncogene

TRANSFECTION

Mouse
Cells

TRANSFORMATION

Foci of Transformed
Cells

CANCER

What Do We Know About the Protein
Products of Protooncogenes?

This is an important aspect of our discussion of oncogenes, an area in which astonishing scientific progress has been made. We now know that the protein products that result from the expression of protooncogenes are involved in an elaborate circuitry that transmits signals from the cell membrane into the nucleus and controls the basic functions of growth, differentiation, and division. Mutations in the protooncogenes may give rise to oncogenes and altered proteins that interfere with this signaling chain and can lead to cancer. Future research in cancer prevention and therapy will focus on finding ways to interfere with these aberrant proteins and their resultant deviant signals. In fact, such experiments targeted at modifying the protein product of the *ras* oncogene are under way in a number of laboratories.

A map localizing the sites of action of some normal protein products appears in figure 3.2, letting the code for each gene stand for its protein product. These encompass a wide array of functions in different regions of the cell. Some proteins are extracellular growth factors; some, located in the membrane, are receptors of growth factors; others are enzymes that transmit and amplify signals from the outside of the cell to the nucleus; one group interacts with protooncogene protein products that are bound to the DNA in the nucleus, and this combination activates or stimulates the expression of other genes.

Extensive studies in experimental mice have helped define the roles of some of these proteins. For example, those that lacked an *int*-1 protooncogene failed to develop a large segment of the brain and died soon after birth. The c-*src* protooncogene was shown to be specifically involved in bone growth, and the c-*kit* gene in the development of bone marrow, gonadal, and pigment-producing cells.

The c-*jun* protooncogene, discovered by Peter Vogt, appears to be a crucial factor in carcinogenesis. It functions as a central switch, receiving signals from growth factors outside the cell and controlling genes in the nucleus that regulate growth and division. An altered c-*jun* (oncogene) acts as a defective switch, relaying inappropriate messages that can lead to unregulated cell growth and cancer. The discovery of *jun* and the *jun-fos* complex has provided an opportunity to analyze cancer induction in the most fundamental manner: at the level of the genome and the control of gene expression.

FIGURE 3.2   Schematic Functions of Protooncogene Protein Products

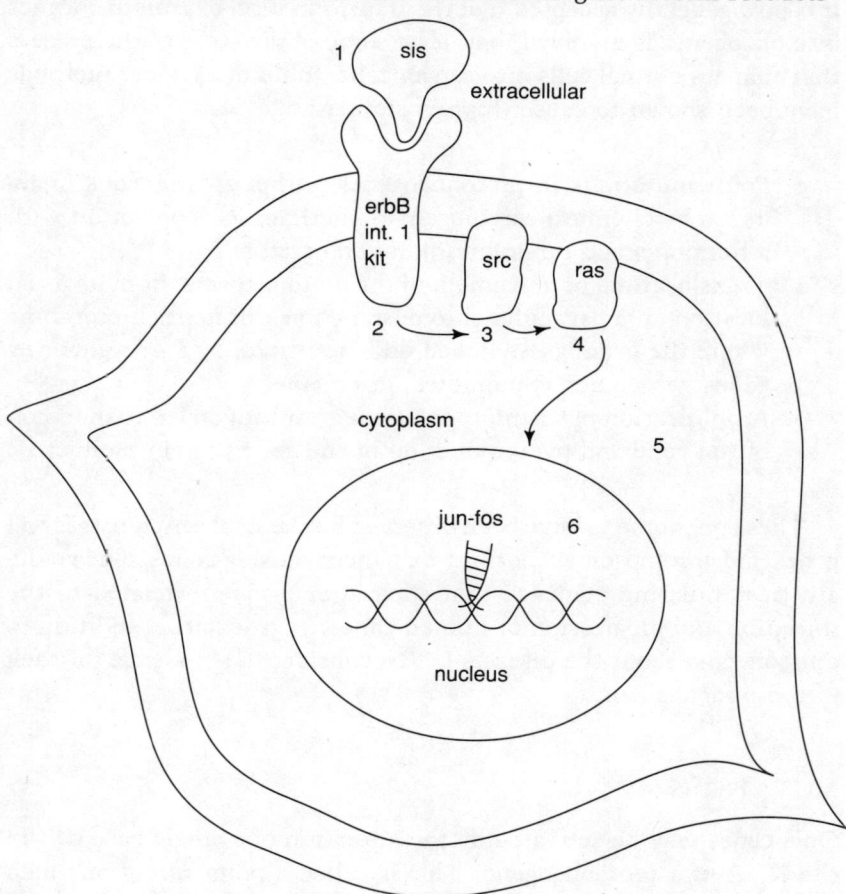

Functions of representative protooncogene protein products in extracellular and cellular compartments. Growth factors (1) bind to and activate cell surface receptors (2), leading to amplification (3) and transduction (4) of second messages (5) through the cytoplasm into the nucleus, where transcription activators (6) lead to gene expression and cell division (mitosis).

How Are Protooncogenes Transformed into Oncogenes?

It is now generally accepted that the transformation of protooncogenes into oncogenes is involved in at least some of the steps of the process that changes normal cells into cancer cells. In humans, three methods have been shown to cause this transformation:

1. Point mutations in protooncogenes, either spontaneous or induced by chemical carcinogens (sometimes in cooperation with a hormone) and other environmental factors.
2. Translocation, or movement of the protooncogene from its usual location on a particular chromosome to a different chromosome where the gene is "switched on" (activated) by its neighboring genes, which act as promoters or enhancers.
3. Amplification of the protooncogene, resulting in overexpression of the gene and overproduction of the gene protein product.

These phenomena have been observed by classical geneticists for all genes and chromosomes, not just for cancer-causing genes. The gradually accumulating evidence that such alterations are related to the initiation and progression of human cancer is an exciting addition to our concepts about the disease. Let us consider the evidence for each of these mechanisms.

MUTATIONS

Oncogenes may be activated by the alteration of a single base pair in the DNA of a protooncogene. This is called a *point mutation.* Such alterations may occur spontaneously in the normal processes of cell division, from the inadvertent deletion of a base, the insertion of an extra base, or the substitution of one base for another. As we have pointed out, there are DNA repair mechanisms that in most cases restore the DNA to its original state. The incidence of such mutations rises with increased cell proliferation, but the question of whether such increased proliferation is not only a necessary but a sufficient condition to explain increased carcinogenesis is unresolved. The current evidence points to cancer in humans as being caused by progressive changes at critical sites in the conversion of normal cells to fully malignant ones.

Point mutations of protooncogenes can also be initiated by chemical carcinogens, for example, nitrosamines and polycyclic aromatic hydrocarbons such as methylcholanthrene and dimethylbenzanthracene. In many cases, these compounds are converted in the body to more reactive species that are, in fact, the initiators of the carcinogenic process. In 1979, Robert Weinberg's group used methylcholanthrene to transform mouse cells into malignant cells. The DNA isolated from these cancer cells could transfect mouse cells, while the DNA from untransformed cells could not. The transforming agent was determined to be the c-*mos* oncogene, providing the first definite link between an oncogene and chemically induced carcinogenesis.

Since those initial studies, two more oncogenes have been shown by transfection techniques to be the transforming agents in chemically induced carcinomas and fibrosarcomas. Additional studies in rats using an array of chemical mutagens (substances that can be shown to cause mutations in DNA) and carcinogens (substances that can cause cancer) also indicated the point mutations in the *ras* oncogenes as the transforming agent. By 1987, investigators at the National Institutes of Health were able to show that consistent point mutations in three c-*ras* protooncogenes yielded oncogenes that were present in many human cancers. The point mutations were identified in specific regions of the *ras* gene, and each resulted in a different amino acid in a particular position in the c-*ras* protein product. Cell transformation was observed within several hours after one such modified *ras* protein product was injected into normal human cells or mouse cells, pinpointing the protein as the crucial agent.

Scientists have learned that approximately 20 percent of all human cancers, including the big three killers—lung, colon, and pancreatic—are, at least in part, brought about by mutations in the *ras* gene whose protein product is critical in cell-signaling pathways. When the mutant product replaces the normal protein in the membrane of a transformed cell, an important switch in a metabolic pathway localized in the cell membrane fails to shut off, leading to the uncontrolled proliferation of cells, one step along the road to the development of cancer.

Only a short time ago, the prospect of using a therapeutic strategy to interfere with the action of the aberrant protein would have seemed remote. In the last few years, however, an interesting line of research has developed that brings this prospect much closer. Recent work in a number of laboratories has revealed that in order for the *ras* protein to become embedded in the cell membrane to perform its function, it must first acquire a lipid or fat tail. The hope now is that it may be possible to interfere with this combination of the carcinogenic protein and the fat tail and prevent one step in the multistep transformation that leads to cancer. It has already been demonstrated that if yeast or animal cells are inoculated with compounds that prevent the fat tail from attaching to the *ras* oncogene protein, cell proliferation can be inhibited.

In some animal studies it was found that two events (exposure to both a chemical carcinogen and estrogens) were required for the initiation of breast cancer as well as for the initiation of skin cancer (topical exposure to both a chemical carcinogen and a so-called promoter). Interesting as these observations of the multistep process of carcinogenesis are, care must be exercised in extrapolating them from cancer in rats to cancer in humans.

TRANSLOCATION

As early as 1902 Theodor Boveri suggested that cancer was due to the abnormal chromosomes he observed in cancer cells. Since then many other cytogeneticists, who study the chromosomes and genes of cells, have suggested that changes in the chromosomes of cancer cells provide clues to their origin. An entirely new aspect of oncogenes and cancer was described in late 1982, when a remarkable association was discovered between the chromosome location of human oncogenes and a type of chromosome change. In *translocation,* one segment of a chromosome breaks off and is joined to another chromosome. For example, in human Burkitt's lymphoma cells, translocation of the cellular c-*myc* gene located on chromosome 8 to a position on chromosome 14 has been observed regularly. Of particular significance is the fact that when this gene relocates on chromosome 14, it is positioned near a group of genes that code for the so-called heavy chain of an immunoglobulin gene. These immunoglobulin genes, present in human B-type lymphocytes, are constantly "switched on" by DNA signals in order to synthesize antibodies to particular foreign substances or antigens. This is an essential mechanism for the immune system to respond to and inactivate antigens. Since the translocation puts the c-*myc* gene close or adjacent to this switch signal, it has been postulated that the signal activates the gene. Indeed, in Burkitt's lymphoma cells, a tenfold to twentyfold overexpression of the c-*myc* gene and its protein product is detected.

Similarly, in a few patients with Burkitt's lymphoma, it has been found that the same region of chromosome 8 where the c-*myc* gene is located has been involved in reciprocal translocations with either chromosome 2 or 22, but in these cases the c-*myc* oncogene remains on chromosome 8. It was demonstrated that the translocated segment of chromosome 2 carries the gene for another immunoglobulin, and the segment of chromosome 22, the gene for still another. As a result of the three chromosome translocations reported in Burkitt's lymphoma—chromosomes 8 to 14, 2 to 8, and 22 to 8—the c-*myc* must be released from its normal regulatory machinery on chromosome 8. The *myc* protooncogene is now juxtaposed near one of the three immunoglobulin gene loci and the immunoglobulin enhancer regulatory elements. It is proposed that these enhancers up-regulate the transcription of the c-*myc* oncogene in B-lymphocytes, leading to overproduction of the protein product.

Many leukemias and lymphomas are associated with consistent translocations of protooncogenes (see appendix, table 10). The detailed study of chromosomal aberrations using new cytogenetic techniques has led to the isolation of new oncogenes, to possible new therapies, and to improved diagnosis.

AMPLIFICATION

Cytogeneticists, using special staining techniques, have detected two other chromosomal abnormalities in many human tumors: extra small chromosomes, called double minute chromosomes, and large bands that show up as homogeneously stained regions. These phenomena have been shown to be due to the presence of multiple copies (a tenfold to hundredfold increase) of certain protooncogenes (amplified DNA). Low-level *amplification*, where there are one or two extra copies of a chromosome or a part of a chromosome, is associated with some blood-related cancers (leukemias, lymphomas). In solid tumors, however, greatly increased numbers of the double minute chromosomes are observed; the higher the numbers, the more advanced and aggressive the cancer appears to be.

The c-*myc* gene was the first protooncogene shown to be amplified. Robert Gallo's group at the National Cancer Institute discovered that the cells of a patient with myelocytic leukemia contained eight to thirty copies of c-*myc* gene, which in normal cells is present in only a few copies in each cell. Thereafter, Bishop's group at the University of California, San Francisco, discovered that in a rare form of colon cancer with double minute chromosomes, the c-*myc* protooncogene was amplified to about fifty copies. Since these cancer cells produced fifty times the normal amount of RNA, the result was an increased production of the protein coded for by that gene. (Table 11 in the appendix summarizes those human cancers associated with amplified protooncogenes.)

The detection of multiple copies of oncogenes has had an impact on the clinical management of certain types of cancer. N-*myc* is present in multiple copies in 40 percent of patients with neuroblastoma—a malignant tumor formed of embryonic ganglion cells—and this amplification correlates with advanced stages of the disease and poor prognosis, despite current therapy. Amplification of all members of the *myc* family (c-*myc*, N-*myc*, and L-*myc*) in small-cell lung cancer is also associated with more malignant stages of the disease.

Of special interest is the new information on the c-*erb*B-2 protooncogene (also called *neu* and *HER*-2). Stuart Aaronson and colleagues at the National Cancer Institute discovered that this gene is often amplified and the gene product overexpressed in aggressive human breast cancers. Tests to detect such gene amplification can be used to identify breast cancers with poor prognosis and in planning optimal treatments.

Many tumors are known to carry amplified regions of DNA that contain protooncogenes and magnify their expression. Amplification occurs rarely, if at all, in normal cells but commonly appears, by an as yet unexplained mechanism, as cells progress toward increased malignancy. Detection of amplified protooncogenes currently has a place in the prognosis and clinical management of at least two cancers, breast cancer and neuroblastoma, and may prove useful in others.

Summary of the Role of Oncogenes in Human Cancer

Let us briefly compare the ways oncogenes cause cancer in animals and in humans. In animals, retroviruses that have incorporated oncogenes into their genomes can infect cells and induce cancer after short incubation periods. Retroviruses without oncogenes can infect cells and, when the viral genome is integrated with the host cellular DNA near protooncogenes, can activate the protooncogene and induce cancer. Finally, retroviruses may spontaneously change their location in the cellular DNA and, if they relocate near protooncogenes, lead to activation of the protooncogene.

In human cancer, on the other hand, protooncogenes are transformed to oncogenes, by any of three mechanisms: mutation, chromosomal translocations, or gene amplification. It has been possible to identify a number of oncogenes in human cancers. Members of the *ras* gene family are most common, occurring in at least 20 percent of all human cancers. The *myc* gene family members are also frequently found in human cancers. All Burkitt's lymphomas have c-*myc* oncogenes activated by translocation near immunoglobulin genes. Amplification of c-*myc* and L-*myc*, by an unknown mechanism, in small-cell lung cancers, and of N-*myc* in neuroblastomas is associated with progression to highly malignant tumors. Aggressive breast cancers with poor prognosis have been found to have amplified oncogenes. This gradually accumulating evidence has implicated oncogenes in at least one step in the genesis of human cancers and has expanded our concepts of the disease.

Oncogenes in the Clinical Setting

How do we take the new information about normal protooncogenes and their unruly derivatives, the oncogenes, and use it in tackling day-to-day problems in the doctor's office and in the hospital? Table 12 in the appendix lists the usefulness of detecting oncogene alterations in the diagnosis, prognosis, and treatment of a number of types of cancer. At the moment, such applications are limited, but it seems reasonable to anticipate that laboratory tests for the detection of oncogenes will become more routine, resulting in earlier diagnosis and treatment. Information from such tests may also provide a way of assessing an individual's susceptibility or predisposition to developing cancer.

Other novel strategies are being considered that mount an attack on the protein products of the oncogenes and inhibit cell proliferation. Earlier in the chapter, we discussed the role of some oncogene products as receptors in cell membranes. Specific antibodies to some of these protein receptors have been prepared, and in experiments, *in vitro* and *in vivo*, the antibodies have been shown to curtail the activity of the receptor and cell proliferation. New efforts designed to inhibit the activation of the *ras* family of oncogenes have focused on preventing the incorporation of its protein product, an enzyme, into the cell membrane.

It is hoped that new insights into the mechanism of action of oncogenes and their role in carcinogenesis may afford more ingenious and successful therapies. No therapy directed against a single oncogene, however, is likely to be a magic bullet in view of the multiple factors that lead to cancer. Next we shall direct our attention to the second class of cancer genes, the tumor-suppressor genes.

Chapter 4

Tumor-Suppressor Genes

C ANCER CELLS DIFFER FROM NORMAL CELLS ONLY IN THE ALTERATION of a few crucial genes. Tumor-suppressor genes, the second class of these crucial cancer genes to have been discovered, emerged slowly on the scene in the shadow of the excitement engendered by the discovery of the first class, oncogenes. They are now considered to be as important as, or more important than, oncogenes in the genesis of cancer. If oncogenes are the accelerators of unruly cell growth, their mirror images, the tumor-suppressor genes, are the brakes for such undesirable cell growth.

The two most important tumor-suppressor genes are the Rb gene (for retinoblastoma, an eye cancer) and the p53 gene (named for its protein product, which has a molecular weight of 53,000), the most common mutated gene in human cancer. Most people are born with two normal Rb genes, one from each parent, now known to protect them from retinoblastoma and certain other cancers. For some years, it has also been known that about half the infants or young children in some families do develop retinoblastoma while their siblings do not. All the children in such families inherit one normal gene from one parent and one defective, or missing, gene from the other parent, often the father. If the one healthy gene is damaged by chemicals or radiation (before cells of the retina differentiate, by about age three), tumors will develop in the eyes, often in multiple sites. Children born with two healthy Rb genes will only rarely (about 1 in 40,000 individuals) sustain damage to both Rb genes in the same retinal cell, thereby allowing the tumor or tumors to form. Were the Rb gene linked only to retinoblastoma, it might be considered a curiosity (although an important one, since it gave us insight into damage or loss of each copy of a tumor-suppressor gene). Recently, however, cancer epidemiologists have discovered that children who survive retinoblastoma show a high incidence of bone cancer, osteosarcoma, breast cancer, and small-cell lung cancer. Cells from these tumors are also missing both copies of the Rb gene. (Laboratory studies show that the insertion into osteosarcoma cells of the chromosome 13, which contains the Rb gene, causes the cells to revert to normal. Further, the insertion of even the isolated gene into the sarcoma cells also causes them to be normal.)

Remarkably, the immense impact of the Rb gene on cancer has been outdone by evolving information about another tumor-suppressor gene, p53. This gene has now been implicated as one contributing factor in the development of at least half of all human cancers in the United States and the United Kingdom. In this chapter we will discuss the history and current status of the Rb, p53, and other tumor-suppressor genes, including their role in many inherited as well as noninherited cancers and in cancer treatment.

The theory that cancer could result from alterations in two genetic elements on chromosomes (now identified as oncogenes and tumor-suppressor genes) was first suggested by Theodor Boveri in 1914: "The unlimited tendency to rapid proliferation in malignant tumor cells [could result] from a permanent predominance of the chromosomes that promote division. . . . Another possibility is the presence of definite chromosomes which inhibit division. . . . Cells of tumors with unlimited growth would arise if those inhibiting chromosomes were eliminated. . . . [Since] each kind of chromosome is represented twice in the normal cell, the depression of only one of these two might pass unnoticed" (Boveri 1914).

In accord with the concept of the existence of two sets of cancer genes, the genetic alterations in cancer cells are of two sorts: dominant and recessive. Alterations of normal protooncogenes into oncogenes, described in the previous chapter, lead to a dominant gain of function; that is, change in only *one* of the two copies, or *alleles*, of a protooncogene leads to an uninhibited growth of cells. On the other hand, alterations in tumor-suppressor genes cause a recessive loss of function; that is, *both* alleles must be inactive in order for cell growth to go unchecked. Loss of function of only one of the two alleles would "pass unnoticed," as Boveri suggested.

Therefore, tumor-suppressor genes are also known as *recessive cancer genes* or *antioncogenes*. Although only about twelve tumor-suppressor genes have been positively identified (in contrast to about sixty oncogenes), they are known to be immensely important in the vast majority of human cancers, including 50 percent of breast cancers and perhaps 100 percent of colon cancers. Lesions in protooncogenes and tumor-suppressor genes seem to be equally common in human cancers, but the number of tumor-suppressor genes damaged in an individual cancer may be greater. Most cancers arise from a multistep process in which alterations in dominant oncogenes and recessive tumor-suppressor genes are both involved. Only tumor-suppressor genes appear to be involved in inherited cancers, however.

It took many researchers many years to get us to this point in our knowledge of tumor-suppressor genes (see timeline).

In 1967, over fifty years after Boveri's statement, Elisabeth Gateff and Howard Schneiderman at Case Western Reserve University in Cleveland recognized that a mutation in both copies of a specific gene in drosophila resulted in brain tumors of the larvae. Two years later, Henry Harris at England's Oxford University and George Klein at Sweden's Karolinska Institute would link tumors to the loss of a tumor-suppressor gene. These investigators discovered that the fusion of normal mouse cells with mouse cancer cells resulted in fused, hybrid cells that were not malignant. This suggested that something in the normal cells could suppress the malignant properties of the cancer cells. Further studies indicated that the suppressive activity could be attributed to certain chromosomes contributed by the normal cells in the fusion. The cancer cells seemed to be defective in functions that inhibited the aggressive proliferation of cancer cells.

Even after tumor suppression, however, the capacity to form tumors reappeared after tissue culture passage or growing of several generations of the hybrid cell populations, and, notably, the tumorigenicity was associated with loss of chromosomes from the hybrid cells. This led to the important concept that normal cells contain dominant suppressor genes that down-regulate cancer genes; these suppressor genes are lost during the chromosome loss from the hybrid cells, thus leading to the reexpression of the tumor genes.

The importance of these cell fusion studies was not recognized because at the time much emphasis was being devoted to the virus theory of cancer. Also little noticed at the time was a report, in 1971, by Alfred Knudson of the M. D. Anderson Hospital and Tumor Institute in Houston, Texas, which proposed that retinoblastoma is caused by two mutations. In the same year, Sir Richard Doll and his colleagues at Oxford University concluded, on the basis of their

TIMELINE OF IMPORTANT
RESEARCHERS IN TUMOR-SUPPRESSOR
GENES

1914   Theodor Boveri theorizes that malignant tumor cells could result from the predominance of chromosomes that promote division (now sites of oncogenes) or from the elimination of "inhibiting" chromosomes (now sites of tumor-suppressor genes).

1967   Elisabeth Gateff and Howard Schneiderman recognize that mutation in both copies of a gene leads to a brain cancer in larvae of the fruit fly drosophila (now known that they are the two copies of a tumor-suppressor gene).

1969   Henry Harris and George Klein discover that mouse cancer cells are rendered nonmalignant when fused to normal mouse cells (the normal cells provide tumor-suppressor genes to the cancer cells).

1971   Alfred Knudson proposes that a childhood cancer of the eye is caused by two mutations of genes (these were later proved to be alterations, or loss, of the two copies of the first tumor-suppressor gene to be discovered, Rb).

1974   Vincent Riccardi and Uta Franke discover that Wilms' tumors have a deletion in chromosome 11.

1976   Eric Stanbridge repeats Harris's work, fusing normal and cancerous mouse cells by using normal and cancerous human cells. The fused cells are nonmalignant, suggesting the presence of tumor-suppressor genes in the normal human cells.

1983   Bernard Mechler isolates Gateff's drosophila brain tumor gene. This is the first example of a tumor-suppressor gene.

1986   Eric Stanbridge and Bernard Weissman fuse human chromosome 11 into human cancer cells (HeLa), thereby suppressing their tumor-forming capacity in mice. This indicates the presence of a tumor-suppressor gene on human chromosome 11.

1988   Thaddeus Dryja, Robert Friend, and Robert Weinberg clone the first human tumor-suppressor gene. Mutations, or deletions, of both copies of this gene (Rb) have been associated with eye (retinoblastoma) and bone (osteosarcoma) tumors of children and cancers of the lung, breast, cervix, prostate, and bladder in adults.

1988   Wen-Hwa Lee inserts the Rb gene into cultured retinoblas-
        toma and osteosarcoma cells and converts the cancer cells into
        normal cells.

1989   Arnold Levine, Samuel Benchimol, and Bert Vogelstein dis-
        cover that p53, first thought to be an oncogene, is in its
        unaltered form a tumor-suppressor gene. Loss of function of
        both copies of p53 gene is detected in approximately 50 per-
        cent of human cancers in the United States and the United
        Kingdom.

1990   Francis Collins and Ray White clone the neurofibromatosis
        type 1 gene, NF1, and Bert Vogelstein clones the "deleted in
        colon carcinoma" gene, DCC.

epidemiological studies, that common human cancers result from as
many as two to six separate mutations in their DNA, depending on the
specific type of cancer.

Knudson noted that retinoblastoma occurs in both hereditary (concentrated in certain families) and nonhereditary forms. The former is
less common than the latter, and tends to occur in younger children,
often in both eyes. Knudson's astute analyses of previous reports of
this tumor and of his own patient population led him to conclude that
the hereditary form of retinoblastoma is the result of one inherited
mutation of a gene that is present in either the egg or the sperm cell
of one parent and therefore in all the body cells of the offspring. A
second mutation must occur in the retinal cells after conception but
before the patient's embryonal retinal cells become mature. The nonhereditary form, on the other hand, is caused by two retinal cell
mutations, but both of these occur after conception and before the
patient's retinal cells mature.

Two important concepts surfaced in a paper published by Knudson
in 1971: (1) two mutations are involved in the genesis of retinoblastoma, and (2) cancer and differentiation of cells are intimately related.
In order for the retinal cells to become cancerous, they must have had
two mutations before they become differentiated into mature cells.

Eventually the two mutations in the childhood cancers proposed by
Knudson were discovered by molecular biological studies to be in each
of the two alleles of the prototype tumor-suppressor gene called Rb.
Such studies have also been used to detect a predisposition to retinoblastoma in individual newborn infants who have a mutation in one
of the Rb gene alleles.

Following up on Harris's studies of fusion of mouse cells, Eric Stanbridge, at the University of California, Irvine, in 1976 reported fusion of normal human cells and cancer cells that clearly supported the concept of tumor-suppressor genes in normal human cells. His work suffered as a result of the focus on oncogenes at the time, however, and little attention was paid to his convincing results.

By this time, the late 1970s, results had shown that oncogenes acting either individually, such as the v-src oncogene, or collabora- tively, such as v-myc and v-ras, could produce a cancer cell without requiring the loss or inactivation of putative tumor-suppressor genes. Therefore, the reports of the fruit fly geneticists and of Harris, Klein, Knudson, and Stanbridge went largely unheeded.

In 1983, however, Bernard Mechler, at the German Cancer Re- search Institute in Heidelberg, Germany, cloned (isolated) the first tumor-suppressor gene in drosophila. As described, Gateff had reported in 1967 that mutations in this gene caused brain tumors in the flies' larvae, without recognizing it as a tumor-suppressor gene. Mechler determined that the gene codes for a protein that is synthesized early in embryogenesis and that drosophila with defects in both copies of the gene develop tumors of the brain and die as larvae. When the tumor cells were injected into adult fruit flies, they invaded the host's tissue and killed them after a few days, an obvious demonstration that the cells with defects in both alleles of a tumor-suppressor gene were malignant. Tumor-suppressor genes finally emerged as the second class of cancer genes in 1986, when Stanbridge and Weissman demon- strated by the use of an ingenious microcell technique that fusion of chromosome 11 into Wilms' tumor cells suppresses their tumor-form- ing capacity.

The next important observation in the story of tumor-suppressor genes was made by geneticists studying human chromosomes. Because retinoblastoma was obviously transmitted in certain families in a dominant fashion, occurring in about 1 in 40,000 births, cytogen- eticists began to examine the chromosomes in the tumor cells for abnormalities.

In the early 1960s several groups reported partial deletions in chro- mosome 13 in a few patients with retinoblastoma. By 1974, eight other patients with retinoblastoma were found to have the same dele- tion. It was not clear, however, that the deletion caused the disease, because by 1980 only 24 of approximately 1,200 retinoblastoma pa- tients were shown to have the deletion, which made its likelihood of being seen only approximately 1 of 50 tumors. Further intensive studies by many investigators have indicated that all retinoblastomas in fact had either deleted areas or point mutations in chromosome 13 or were missing the entire chromosome.

Following these observations of the chromosome deletions in some retinoblastoma cells, similar observations were made in another childhood cancer, Wilms' tumor. Vincent Riccardi, along with Uta Franke, used a new technique that distinguished up to 1,500 bands on stained chromosomes. With this technique they localized the deletion on chromosome 11 in Wilms' tumor cells. The next important research finding was the confirmation of Knudson's 1971 hypothesis by the discovery and cloning of the human retinoblastoma gene in 1988 by Thaddeus Dryja, Robert Friend, and Robert Weinberg. The Rb gene became the prototype tumor-suppressor gene and led to the final acceptance of these genes as the second class of cancer genes and major players in human cancer.

While the investigations of the first two tumor-suppressor genes for retinoblastoma and Wilms' tumor discovered in these inherited childhood cancers were unfolding, a new tumor-suppressor gene, p53, was discovered and immediately took center stage because of its role in the majority of cancers in adults. This gene, present on chromosome 17, was first listed not as a tumor-suppressor gene but as an inconsequential oncogene. It was reported, by Arnold Levine at Princeton University and by other groups in 1979, to be a dominant oncogene because it could immortalize cells in culture. Further studies by Levine and other groups, including Samuel Benchimol at the Ontario Cancer Institute and Bert Vogelstein at Johns Hopkins University, showed that when one copy of the gene was mutated it functioned as an oncogene but that both copies of the p53 gene were altered in certain cancer tissues, suggesting that it was a recessive tumor-suppressor gene.

That made p53 a "hermaphrodite" gene. When one copy of the gene is mutated it acts as an oncogene in laboratory studies, but when both copies are mutated, or deleted, various cancers can develop. Thus when both normal (wild type) copies (alleles) of the gene are functioning, they suppress tumor formation.

What Do Tumor-Suppressor Genes Do?

Evidence is now emerging indicating that tumor-suppressor genes act as regulatory genes that control the expression of other genes. Such regulatory genes have been well studied in bacteria. For instance, in the bacillus *E. coli,* repressor genes code for proteins that bind to specific sequences of the bacterial DNA and block access of the RNA polymerase enzyme to particular genes. The repressor proteins thus block transcription and the synthesis of the protein products of those particular genes. Besides such genes for negative or down-regulation, bacteria also have positive regulatory genes that code for gene activation proteins. These proteins bind to DNA and facilitate the binding of RNA polymerase and subsequent transcription of a gene product. Such a positive or up-regulatory gene would be similar to the oncogene *jun* discussed in chapter 3.

In multicellular organisms, very little is known about the genes that down-regulate other genes. In fact, the discovery of tumor-suppressor genes has added much new information about them. It is theorized that during the cellular proliferation and differentiation that occur during growth and development of complex multicellular organisms, large numbers of genes must be switched on and off in an orderly way. Studies of the fruit fly drosophila have indicated that alteration (or mutation) of certain genes can convert one part of the body into another (disrupt differentiation). For instance, a mutation of a gene that normally causes a set of cells to form an antenna on the fly's head produces an altered gene that causes the cells to make, instead of an antenna, a leg that grows out of the head. Such observations that alteration of a single gene product can lead to formation of a complex alternative structure have led to the concept that perhaps a small number of master regulator genes, known as *homeotic genes,* and their protein products can orchestrate the development of different major components of complex multicellular organisms. Indeed, the fact that characteristic elements believed important in the control of homeotic genes are well conserved among different animal species tends to support this concept. It is now known that alterations of tumor-suppressor genes, a class of regulator genes, lead to the generation of cells that grow in an unrestrained fashion and cause cancer.

What is known about the genes that act as regulators of expression of retroviral genes and oncogenes, two groups of genes implicated in the origin and proliferation of cancer?

Robert Huebner and George Todaro proposed the existence of regulatory genes, whose gene products provide a "repressor system" for retroviral genes and oncogenes. The general concepts of this hypothesis may eventually prove to be correct. Convincing evidence has been presented by a number of investigators that supports the existence of genetic regulation of retroviral genes in such diverse species as chickens, inbred strains of mice, and wild mice.

Based upon the oncogene theory of Huebner and Todaro and the "two mutation" theory of Knudson, David Comings as early as 1973 proposed a general theory of carcinogenesis. He suggested that all cells contain transforming genes (some of which could be oncogenes), and these, when active, release the cell from its normal constraints on growth. Comings postulated that these genes were normally active during embryogenesis, but that in the process of differentiation they were "turned off" by diploid pairs of regulatory genes. He proposed that a mutation in both alleles of regulatory genes accounted for release of suppression and subsequent transformation of the cell. Only very recently has a body of evidence appeared in support of Comings's proposal.

What Is Known About Regulator Genes for Cancer?

The initial clues about the existence, the anatomy, the chromosomal location, the protein products, and the normal function of tumor-suppressor genes come from studies of the fruit fly. Mutations in 25 of the fruit fly's 5,000 genes are causally related to the development of benign or malignant tumors. In the normal fly, these 25 genes seem to play important roles in the differentiation of specific cell types and tissues. It is not known how many of these 25 genes have sequences homologous to oncogenes and how many may be regulatory or tumor-suppressor genes. However, the homologues of six retroviral oncogenes have been detected in drosophila DNA. At least two drosophila genes have been shown to be recessive-regulator or tumor-suppressor genes. Deficiency or absence of the gene products of one of these genes appears to allow the development of nerve tumors, neuroblastomas, and deficiencies of the other gene that can result in brain and retinal tumors. It is noteworthy that, in addition to these two genes, the other 23 mutant genes are also recessive, suggesting that they are regulatory or suppressor genes that downregulate tumor formation rather than the dominant oncogenes whose increased or altered expression leads to tumor formation.

Interestingly, a homologue of one of these drosophila genes has been detected in human DNA. It will be of great interest to determine whether it can down-regulate the N-*myc* oncogene that is over-expressed in neuroblastoma and retinoblastoma cells and cause the reversion of these cancer cells to a normal phenotype. Further, how many of the 25 drosophila suppressor genes will be detected in the human genome, and what is their relationship to cancer?

Tumor-Suppressor Genes in Childhood Cancer

Knudson quickly expanded his astute observations about retinoblastoma—that it occurred in a familial or hereditary form in infants and very young children, often seen in both eyes as multiple tumors (40 percent of cases), and in a sporadic, nonhereditary form in older children, seen as a single tumor in only one eye (60 percent of cases)—to two other childhood cancers: Wilms' tumor of the kidney and neuroblastoma, a cancer of nerve ectodermal cells. Both occurred as either hereditary, bilateral tumors (for instance, Wilms' tumors in both kidneys) in young children or as nonhereditary, unilateral tumors in older children. These observations led to the discovery of the first two tumor-suppressor genes, the Rb gene of retinoblastoma and the WT gene of Wilms' tumor.

The Rb gene was discovered first. This was based on the observation that a small fraction of the cases, about 3 percent, demonstrate a deletion of chromosome 13 in both the tumor cells and the normal cells. Some of these deletions are very large and others are small, but all include one band, 13q14, that usually appears after staining on chromosome 13. ("Stained" chromosomes show dark bands.) It was surmised that this missing band is the site of the antiretinoblastoma tumor-suppressor gene. It was also realized that this proposed site of the Rb gene is near the site of an already known gene that codes for the enzyme esterase D.

Robert Sparks of UCLA, along with William Benedict and Linn Murphree at the University of Southern California Childrens Hospital in Los Angeles, used the information that the putative Rb gene and esterase D gene are closely linked on chromosome 13 to conduct a series of ingenious experiments using esterase D protein as a "marker." These were based on the findings that when one copy of the esterase D gene is deleted, the esterase D level is 50 percent of the normal amount detected when both genes are present. Using this information, the group then studied the normal tissues and tumor tissues of patients with hereditary (bilateral) and nonhereditary (unilateral) retinoblastoma. The exciting results indicated that patients with hereditary retinoblastoma and chromosome 13q14 deletions had 50 percent esterase D levels in their normal cells (indicating one esterase D gene and one Rb gene missing) but 0 esterase D levels in their tumor cells (indicating both esterase D and both Rb genes missing). Patients with nonhereditary retinoblastomas had normal esterase D levels in their normal cells but 0 levels in their tumor cells. These observations supported Knudson's concepts and suggested that the loss of both copies of a tumor-suppressor gene results in a tumor of retinal cells. Those patients with hereditary tumors were born with only one normal Rb and esterase D allele and lost the activity of that normal allele in their tumors after birth. Those with nonhereditary tumors were born with two normal alleles but subsequently lost them both and developed retinal tumors. Thus infants with hereditary loss of one Rb allele were at greater risk of losing the second allele (in the same retinal cell) at an earlier age and in more retinal cells than those infants who began life with two normal copies of the Rb gene. These conclusions fit with observations that infants with hereditary retinoblastomas develop the tumors at a younger age and in multiple sites, while those with nonhereditary tumors have only one tumor that forms at an older age.

The suppressor genes that regulate retinoblastoma may also play a role in suppressing the development of other malignancies. For instance, children who survive hereditary retinoblastoma (who are born with one allele of the pair of suppressor alleles of the Rb gene already mutated or inactive) develop bone tumors, osteosarcomas, two thousand times more frequently in the skull and five hundred times more frequently in the extremities than would be expected in the general population. For instance, 15 percent of bilateral retinoblastomas develop osteosarcomas in bones that were not exposed to X rays used to treat the tumor (and therefore clearly not caused by the X-ray treatment). In these cases, the view is that one Rb allele is altered in all the patient's body cells, inherited from a parent's defective egg or sperm cell (first "hit"), and the other allele is altered in the primitive bone cells or osteoblasts (second "hit"). In sporadic osteosarcomas, both "hits" apparently occur in the same osteoblast after conception. Another study revealed that in addition to the high incidence of osteosarcomas, 40 percent of individuals who survived hereditary retinoblastoma were dead from a second primary malignancy of various types within thirty years after diagnosis of the retinoblastoma.

The tissue specificity exhibited by the Rb gene has been called remarkable and mysterious. The gene product is widely expressed in many tissues, yet the inherited defect in one of the normal copies of the gene appears to create a predisposition to tumors of only two types, retinoblastoma and osteosarcoma. In contrast, when both copies of the gene are originally normal but both are damaged later in life, a wide variety of cancers may result. These observations indicate that the retinoblastoma regulatory gene plays an important role in regulating cancers other than retinoblastoma. Recent evidence, in fact, suggests that the Rb gene also suppresses certain breast, prostate, bladder, cervical, ovarian, and small-cell lung cancers.

Besides retinoblastoma, Wilms' tumor, a kidney cancer of children, occurs in hereditary and nonhereditary forms, and the statistical analysis of the age of occurrence fits the Knudson two-hit hypothesis, namely, the hereditary form occurs at a younger age than the nonhereditary. This tumor has been associated with similar chromosomal changes to those noted in retinoblastoma. In Wilms' tumors, the changes, seen in both hereditary and nonhereditary forms, apparently consist of deletions or inactivations of band p13 of chromosome 11 or loss of one chromosome 11 (in retinoblastoma, it is chromosome 13 that has the changes). These gross chromosomal changes are present in the tumor tissue of 55 percent of Wilms' tumor patients; they are not seen in noncancerous tissues of the same patients. In the other 45 percent, it is proposed that smaller changes in the same band of chromosome 11 are present but cannot be detected by current methods.

As in retinoblastoma, these changes may be viewed as a loss or an inactivation of both alleles of the gene, leading to the formation of Wilms' tumors. In the hereditary form, one hit has occurred in the germ cell line, and the other occurs after conception in an immature kidney cell. In the nonhereditary, sporadic form, both hits occur in the same immature kidney cell. As in patients with retinoblastoma who also develop osteosarcomas, Wilms' tumor patients develop two other embryonal tumors, rhabdomyosarcomas (tumors of muscle cells) and hepatoblastomas (tumors of liver cells) that appear to be related to the inactivation of the genes on chromosome 11. The regulatory gene for embryonal rhabdomyosarcoma, however, has been determined to be distinct from the Wilms' tumor gene, being located at a separate site on chromosome 11.

Still another example of a childhood embryonal cancer possibly associated with loss or inactivation of a regulatory gene is neuroblastoma, a tumor of nerve cells. Statistical analysis of its occurrence fits the two-hit hypothesis applied to retinoblastomas and Wilms' tumors, and a significant number of tumors have a deletion of a specific area at the end of the short arm of chromosome 1.

Besides these initial examples of the loss of regulatory genes in the pathogenesis of six embryonal tumors—retinoblastoma, osteosarcoma, Wilms' tumor, rhabdomyosarcoma, hepatoblastoma, and neuroblastoma—examples of similar deletions of genes have been reported in tumors of adults.

Tumor-Suppressor Genes in Adult Cancer

Childhood tumors comprise only a minor segment of cancer cases— $\pm$ 6,000 new cases in the United States every year, compared with $\pm$ 1,040,000 new cases of serious cancer (excluding skin) among adults per year (DeVita et al. 1989, p. 296)—and it was important to learn whether tumor-suppressor genes were also major factors in the development of adult cancers.

For years cytogeneticists pointed out that, while chromosomal translocations were often seen in leukemias and lymphomas, chromosomal deletions were common in solid tumors of adults. The first example of deletions in adult cancer being associated with tumor-suppressor genes were those seen in nerve-cell tumors of the adult nervous system.

A number of workers reported the loss of genetic markers on chromosome 22 associated with the development of acoustic neuromas, tumors of the hearing nerve. These tumors, like retinoblastoma, Wilms' tumors, and neuroblastomas, occur in familial, bilateral forms and noninherited, unilateral forms. These findings suggest that the loss of both copies of a tumor-suppressor gene on chromosome 22 may play a significant role in acoustic neuromas.

Another cancer of adults, familial renal-cell (kidney) carcinoma, again follows the retinoblastoma pattern in that the hereditary form occurs at an earlier age than the nonhereditary form and tends to develop in both kidneys. In this tumor, the translocation of chromosomal segments between chromosomes 3 and 8 suggested a mutation or deletion at the breaking points where the translocations occur. Follow-up studies have, in fact, indicated loss of alleles on chromosome 3.

Similarly, in small-cell lung cancer, specific deletions on chromosome 3 have been observed, and in multiple endocrine neoplasia type

2, deletions on chromosome 1 were discovered. Other studies of transitional-cell bladder carcinoma have detected deletions on chromosome 11.

Finally, two groups have reported deletion of a suppressor gene called APC, for adenomatous polyposis cole, on chromosome 5 in a type of colon cancer, dominant familial adenomatous polyposis (APC). The benign polyps that form in the colon of these patients appear to have lost only one allele of the FAP-suppressor gene, while the malignant cancer cells that often develop in these polyps have lost both alleles.

Thus, in addition to six embryonal tumors of children, a number of cancers of adults (listed in appendix, table 13) have chromosomal deletions suggesting that the loss of tumor-suppressor genes may be a step leading to the final appearance of a malignant cancer cell. From these observations it would appear that the human genome may contain many tumor-suppressor genes, perhaps equal to or more than the number of oncogenes. Defective or missing alleles of these suppressor genes might lead to the formation of solid tumors in different tissues.

Following these initial observations about chromosome deletions in various adult cancers, the startling discovery was made that the p53 gene, originally thought (in 1979) to be an oncogene, was in its unmutated form the most important tumor-suppressor gene for the majority of human tumors. Groups at the Ontario Cancer Institute and Johns Hopkins University discovered in 1989 that both copies of the p53 gene were altered, often mutated or deleted, in various cancers. Some mutations were spontaneous, and others were caused by environmental carcinogens. For instance, liver tumors in patients from geographic areas where hepatitis B virus and aflatoxin are causative factors had mutations in one specific site in the p53 gene (codon 249). Evidence now suggests that the role of the p53 tumor-suppressor gene is similar to that of the Rb gene in that it generally fits the two-hit model of Knudson: both alleles of the gene must be rendered inactive, or deleted, in order for a cancer to develop.

The usual function of the p53 gene is to suppress proliferation of normal cells. Each cell has two copies, alleles, of the p53 gene. If one copy is normal (designated "wild") and the other altered (mutated) so that it is not fully active or expressed, the gene can still control growth and suppress cancer development. If both copies of the p53 gene are inactivated, the cell can escape from the suppression of growth and a cancer can develop. This p53 gene, located on chromosome 17p, is the tumor-suppressor gene most commonly associated with human cancers: breast, colon, lung, liver, esophagus, brain, adrenal-gland, and leukemias and sarcomas.

As with the Rb gene, some of the mutations in one copy of the p53 gene occur in germ cells and therefore can be inherited. One possible example of a mutated p53 gene is one that leads to familial breast cancer that usually occurs in young women. In this example, the one inherited mutant allele of the p53 gene is the "initiating event," and subsequent events, such as the inactivation of the normal gene allele and activation of oncogenes, eventually lead to development of breast cancer.

As noted earlier, families who have one defective tumor-suppressor Rb gene have a high incidence of retinoblastoma. Similarly, about 100 families with one mutated p53 gene have now been identified; the various cancers observed to occur in these families have been designated the Li-Fraumeni syndrome (named for the work of Frederick Li and Joseph Fraumeni).

In families devastated by the Li-Fraumeni syndrome, the inherited p53 gene mutations on chromosome 17p usually consist of loss of one copy of the gene and later a point mutation in the other copy. The total accumulation of later events, especially exposure to carcinogens, including ionizing irradiation, leads to a variety of fibrous and epithelial tumors at different sites. Patients with the inherited gene defect usually develop cancer in about ten to thirty years. In contrast to the Li-Fraumeni families who have an inherited p53 gene defect and early-onset cancers, individuals in the general population who do not have a familial p53 gene defect usually develop cancer late in life. In these cancers, although defects in the p53 gene are commonly present, it appears to be a late event in the progression toward cancer. For instance, in colon and rectal cancers most p53 mutations occur late in the progression to the malignant state and are not detected in premalignant adenomas (see chapter 5).

The interesting saga of the p53 tumor-suppressor gene could eventually lead to public health screening for the defective gene. If a mutated or missing copy of the gene is detected in female babies, it would be important for them to obtain mammograms before the currently recommended forty years of age, for example.

Besides p53, two more genes have been discovered that suppress adult cancers. In 1990, Francis Collins at the University of Michigan and Ray White at the University of Utah reported that they had isolated the neurofibromatosis type 1 gene (NF1). An interesting gene dose effect is associated with this tumor-suppressor gene, located on chromosome 17. Mutations in *one* copy of the NF1 gene result in neurofibromatosis, also known as von Recklinghausen's disease. This is a hereditary disorder consisting of pigmented spots and benign tumors of the skin and nerves, as well as bony deformities. Defects in *both* copies of this gene may lead to malignant neurofibrosarcomas and an increased risk of other malignancies.

Also in 1990, Vogelstein discovered another tumor-suppressor gene, located on chromosome 18. The gene has been named DCC because it is *d*eleted in *c*olon *c*arcinomas (that is, it can no longer be detected by staining the chromosome). Such deletions, along with alterations in oncogenes and other tumor-suppressor genes, are one of the multiple steps leading to colon cancer.

The ever-growing family of tumor-suppressor genes clearly played significant roles in both childhood and adult cancers.

What Is the Structure of Tumor-Suppressor Genes, and How Do Their Products Govern Cancer-Cell Proliferation?

These questions are answered best for the Rb and p53 genes. The Rb gene, cloned by Thaddeus Dryja at the Massachusetts Eye and Ear Infirmary, is located on chromosome 13 at the q14 band. It spreads over more than 200,000 base pairs of DNA and consists of 27 exons (expressed regions of DNA) that are transcribed into 4,700-base pairs in RNA. The Rb protein has a molecular weight of 105,000 (and this would be designated p105). It is present in cells of all tissues and in all phases of the cell cycle. Even when the protein from only one copy of the Rb gene is present, it restrains cell growth in normal cells. When both copies of the gene are inactivated or missing, however, the cells proliferate and tumors can develop in specific tissues (see figure 4.1). The Rb gene has been clearly shown to function as a suppressor of tumor formation. In 1988, Wen-Hwa Lee and colleagues at the University of California at San Diego inserted the Rb gene into the retinoblastoma and osteosarcoma cells and showed that the Rb-expressing cells could no longer form tumors in mice (see figure 4.2).

It is still not known how the Rb protein stops cell proliferation of normal cells. Some researchers think it binds directly to DNA and down-regulates the transcription of growth-promoting genes. Others

FIGURE 4.1   Models for Rb Activity

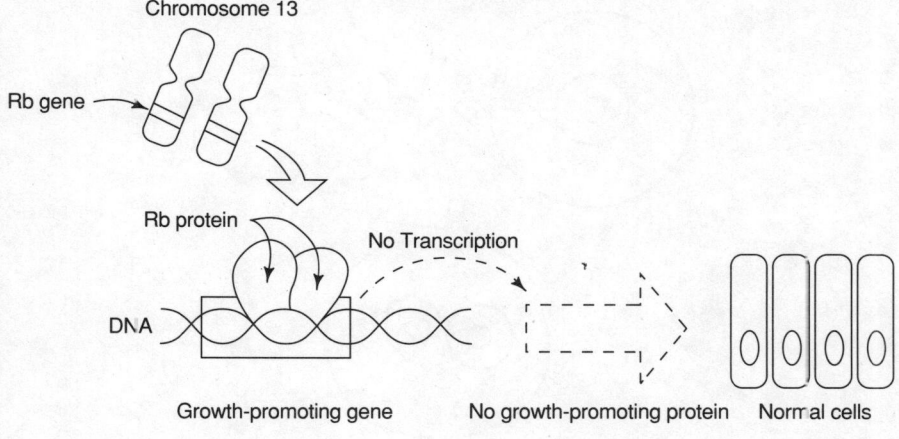

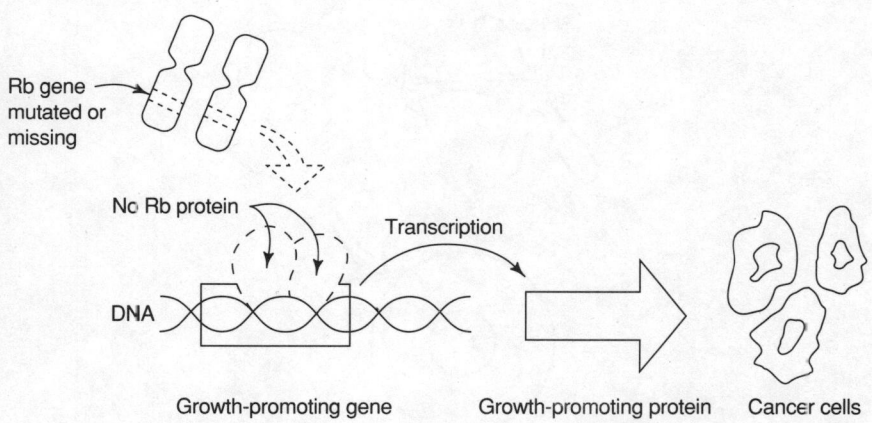

note that Rb activity depends on its phosphorylation state (how many phosphate groups are attached) during the cell cycle. It was found that the protein has few attached phosphate groups early in the cell cycle but many attached groups when DNA is synthesized. Still others point out that the normal Rb protein complexes with, and neutralizes the action of, other growth-promoting proteins, including those of various DNA tumor viruses; SV40, adenoviruses, and papillomaviruses. Many groups are seeking answers to the important question of how the Rb gene controls the proliferation of cancer cells.

FIGURE 4.2

Tumor-suppressor genes in normal cells (A), in chromosomes (B), or as isolated single genes (C) can convert cancer cells into normal cells.

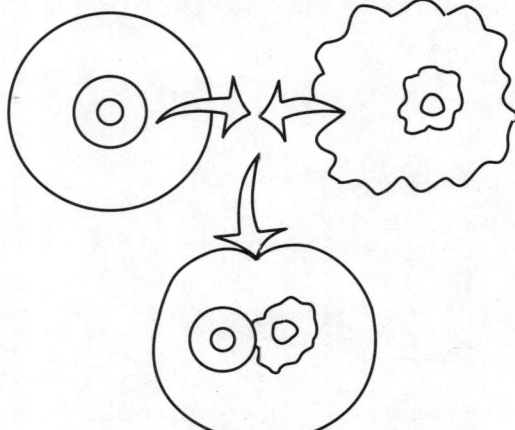

A.   Henry Harris fused a normal cell with a cancer cell. The hybrid cell with two sets of chromosomes was converted into a normal cell.

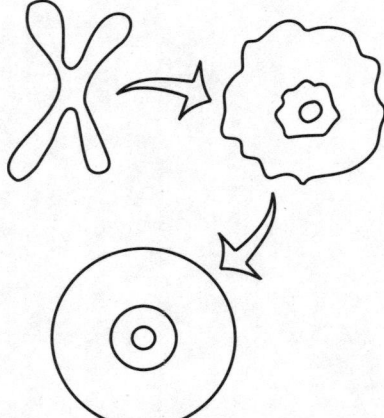

B.   Bernard Weissman and Eric Stanbridge fused a single chromosome from a normal cell into a cancer cell, thereby converting it into a normal cell.

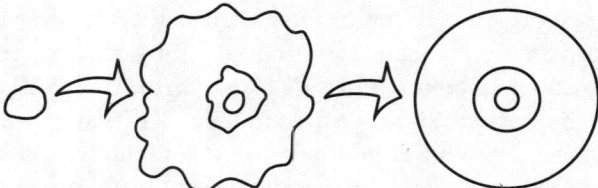

C.   Wen-Hwa Lee inserted a single tumor-suppressor gene into a cancer cell, thereby converting it into a normal cell.

Investigators are also studying the function of the p53 gene. It was cloned by Arnold Levine of Princeton University and others and is comprised of 1,179 base pairs that code for a protein of 53,000 molecular weight (thus the name *p53*). The original gene clones were able to immortalize cells or, in cooperation with the *ras* oncogene, to transform cells. Therefore p53 was considered to be an oncogene. However, all of these transforming p53 gene clones turned out to be mutant forms of the normal ("wild") p53 gene. Thereafter, the unaltered p53 gene was discovered, like the Rb gene, to down-regulate cell growth and division. The normal p53 gene can suppress the growth of transformed cells in culture and the tumor-forming capacity of cancer cells inoculated into animals. Also, like Rb, mutations or deletions of wild-type p53 occur in human tumors. Unlike Rb, however, mutant forms of p53 gain a function so as to stimulate cell division. Two hypotheses have been proposed to explain the function of the normal p53 gene. One states that the p53 binds to DNA and down-regulates the synthesis of DNA in the S phase (DNA synthesis phase) of the cell cycle. Alternatively, the p53 protein, after binding to DNA, down-regulates the transcriptions of genes that effect the passage from G^1 to S phase of the cell cycle. Further studies should determine which of these concepts is correct.

Less is known about the functions of the other tumor-suppressor genes we have mentioned, although the Wilms' tumor gene (WT1), the disseminated colon cancer gene (DCC), and the neurofibromatosis type 1 gene (NF1) have been cloned. The WT1 gene product is expressed in tissues of the developing kidney and apparently functions in normal kidney differentiation. Recent evidence obtained by Stephen Madden and his group at the Wistar Institute of Anatomy and Biology in Philadelphia indicates that the WT1 gene product usually binds to DNA and blocks the transcription of other genes. The gene is mutated or missing in some Wilms' tumors, however—a defect that is associated with unrestrained growth of undifferentiated kidney cells.

At present, it appears that tumor-suppressor genes are universal ingredients of carcinogenesis, whose major functions are likely to be those that govern cell replication and differentiation.

Do Tumor-Suppressor Genes Down-regulate Oncogenes?

The question of central importance to the current interest in onco-genes and tumor-suppressor genes, such crucial elements in the origin of cancer, is whether specific suppressor genes can down-regulate the expression of specific oncogenes in cancer cells. Many observers de-bunk the notion of an antioncogene, but evidence is evolving that it may be closer to the truth than expected.

Some cell-fusion studies by Carlo Croce at the Wistar Institute in Philadelphia in the early 1980s suggested that putative regulatory genes in both mouse NIH 3T3 cells and human lymphoid tumor cells can switch off the transcription of the c-*myc* oncogene in Burkitt's lymphoma cells. Other cell-fusion studies by Eric Stanbridge and Ber-nard Weissman indicated that fusion of normal human fibroblasts to human sarcoma cells rendered the cancer cells nontumorigenic in mice but did not suppress the high levels of the N-*ras* oncogene RNA in the cancer cells. Thus, at least one oncogene was not suppressed by tumor-suppressor gene in normal fibroblasts.

More recent, somewhat fragmentary results show that the Rb gene can reduce the transcription of the c-*myc* protooncogene and suppress the proliferation of skin cells. Also, when a putative tumor-suppressor gene located on chromosome 1 is deleted in human neuroblastoma cells, the N-*myc* oncogene is amplified; further study is needed to determine the significance of this result. Finally, the NF1 tumor-suppressor gene encodes a protein that appears to exercise negative control over one or more of the *ras* oncogenes.

Although the concept of antioncogenes remains mostly theoretical and unproven, many perhaps coincidental examples of alterations of both classes of cancer genes are being found in many human cancers (listed in appendix, table 14).

Tumor-Suppressor Genes in the Clinical Setting

Laboratory detection of the absence of, or damage to, one copy of tumor-suppressor genes, such as Rb, WT1, and p53, is of immense predictive value for an individual's predisposition to retinoblastoma,

Wilms' tumor, Li-Fraumeni syndrome, and other cancers. Other studies can be used to determine the course of the disease. For instance, the greater the number of genetic abnormalities in the FAP, DDC, or p53 gene, the poorer the prognosis of colon or rectal cancer. Molecular diagnostic tests to reveal such abnormalities could serve as a basis for prognosis, selection of optimal therapy, or even prevention by treating premalignant cells.

The multiple genetic lesions in both protooncogenes and tumor-suppressor genes found in most cancers make the concept of gene therapy unrealistic, but there is some hope that not all of the lesions to genes in an individual tumor need to be repaired to achieve some benefit. For instance, in laboratory studies already discussed, the replacement of a single tumor-suppressor gene, Rb, WT1, or p53, has caused several types of cancer cells to revert to normal.

Looking to the future, molecular diagnostic studies of both oncogenes and tumor-suppressor genes will be of immense value in establishing the diagnosis and prognosis of various cancers. Tumor-suppressor genes will also be of great use in determining an individual's predisposition to certain cancers, and they, or their gene products, may prove useful in cancer therapy.

We now move to the very important topic of metastasis.

Chapter 5

Metastasis

S ECONDARY, OR METASTATIC, TUMORS HAVE BEEN KNOWN TO PATIENTS and physicians for centuries. Four hundred years ago, Wilhelm Fabry von Hilden (1560–1624), often called the father of German surgery, "operated for selected carcinoma of the breast and described removal of axillary metastases" (in Shimkin 1977, p. 63). In the nineteenth century, the French physician Joseph Claude Anselme Recamier was the first to recognize how cancer spreads, describing invasions of veins and secondary growth in the brains of patients with breast cancer. He called the process by which the primary cancer had spread to a distant site *metastasis*, from the Greek *meta*, which means "after," "beyond," or "over," and *stasis*, meaning "to stand"—indicating that the cancer had spread from its original location to another stationary location.

An article in a recent scientific journal stated that "the most life-threatening aspect of cancer is the undetected spread of tumor cells throughout the body" (Liotta 1992, p. 54). Indeed, metastases are associated with most treatment failures in cancer patients today. Unfortunately, by the time a primary tumor is diagnosed, about 30 percent of patients already have clinically detectable metastases. Of the other 70 percent, about half have small, undetectable metastases that will appear later. Widely disseminated tumor cells may lie dormant for years before producing fresh crops of metastic tumors. All told, at the time of the initial diagnosis of a solid cancer, about 65 percent of patients already have either clinically detectable or microscopic metastatic tumors (DeVita 1989, p. 98).

The distress and fear of a patient learning of metastasis are well founded. Despite important improvements in early diagnosis, surgical and radiation therapy, and chemotherapy, most cancer complications and deaths are caused by metastases. Innovative strategies to treat metastases are desperately needed, and, indeed, some are on the horizon. Before discussing the process of metastasis, let's review how a normal cell develops into a cancer cell.

How Does a Normal Cell Evolve into a Cancer Cell?

As we have discussed in previous chapters, an individual unruly cell that has escaped the normal regulatory control mechanisms is the basic unit of cancer. A normal, or apparently normal, cell evolves slowly into a cancer cell by means of a sequential accumulation of alterations in the genetic material (DNA) that comprises its protooncogenes and tumor-suppressor genes. Because it takes time for these alterations or mutations to occur, most cancers occur in older people. Cancer incidence increases rapidly with age, especially in individuals over sixty-five.

Some cancers, however, do occur in young adults, infants, and children. On rare occasions a baby is even born with cancer. In many such young patients, their apparently normal cells have one copy of a defective (or missing) tumor-suppressor gene that was inherited from one of their parents. Therefore, fewer total alterations are required for the apparently normal cell to evolve into a cancer cell. These alterations can be caused by spontaneous internal events or by external environmental factors, as illustrated in table 5.1.

The spontaneous internal alterations in protooncogenes are mutations of the genes' DNA, insertions of retroviral DNA, "jumping genes" near the protooncogenes, translocation of a protooncogene near a "turned-on" immunoglobulin gene, or spontaneous amplification of the protooncogene. All of these events can "turn on" or reactivate silent protooncogenes without input from external environmental factors. Similarly, spontaneous internal alterations can occur in tumor-suppressor genes and "turn off" their growth-suppressor actions. These events can be mutations or deletions of the genes, or loss of an entire chromosome containing the gene.

Besides these spontaneous alterations in the two classes of cancer genes, other alterations can be induced by external factors in the environment, such as tobacco or other chemical carcinogens, dietary

TABLE 5.1   *Genesis of Cancer: Effects of Internal and External Factors on Protooncogenes and Tumor-Suppressor Genes*

Protooncogenes (developmental genes, tumor-promotor genes)	1. Normally active during embryogenesis and early childhood, and also discrete phases of the cell cycle thereafter are suppressed by regulatory genes (tumor-suppressor genes).
	2. Reactivated by internal factors: * Endogenous mutations * Relocation of retroviral LTR/promoter/enhancers near protooncogenes * Translocation of protooncogene near immunoglobulin gene * Amplification of protooncogene
	3. Reactivated by external factors: * Chemical carcinogen–induced mutations * Electromagnetic energy: X rays, sunlight * Particulate energy: atomic explosion * Viruses: papillomaviruses, hepatitis, retroviruses * Exogenous factors, for example, hormones
Tumor-Suppressor Genes (antioncogenes)	1. Normally active to suppress protooncogene function after embryogenesis and early childhood.
	2. Inactivated by internal factors: * One copy of the gene may be missing in germ cell * Mutation * Deletion from chromosomal DNA

---

* Loss of chromosome
* Relocation of retroviral DNA into gene
3. Inactivated by external factors:
   * Chemical carcinogens
   * Electromagnetic energy
   * Particulate energy

---

factors, X rays, ultraviolet radiation, viruses, and hormones. The most precise information about the role of these external factors in altering genes is for aflatoxin and sunlight. Aflatoxin, from a mold in food, plays an important role in liver cancers in Asia and Africa by causing a mutation at a specific site (codon 249) in the p53 tumor-suppressor gene. Sunlight plays a specific role in the genesis of skin cancer. The 300 nm wavelength of ultraviolet light causes disruption in the thymidine bases, building blocks of the DNA, at many sites in the cellular DNA, including the p53 tumor-suppressor gene.

From these considerations, a number of conceptual models for the multistep events that allow a normal cell to evolve into a cancer cell have become evident. These are illustrated in table 5.2. Models with as few as two steps are presented for childhood cancers, while those with four or more steps describe adult cancers. The last model in the table, colon cancer, is perhaps the best-studied malignancy in terms of the steps associated with its progression. Bert Vogelstein and colleagues have documented the stepwise progression of colon and rectal cancer: from increased cellular growth, to small benign tumor, to local cancer, to metastasis. It has been possible to obtain tissues that represent these various stages of progression from the same patient and to test the DNA from these tissues for activated oncogenes and inactivation or deletion of tumor-suppressor genes. These studies indicate that at least four of the six steps predicted by epidemiologists can be identified. Thus a case could be made for the role of an activation of protooncogenes c-K-*ras* and c-*myc* and the loss of tumor-suppressor genes on chromosomes 5, 17 (p53), and 18 (DCC) in this cancer. In fact, the *ras* gene is activated in about 50 percent of colon and rectal adenomas, and the regions containing the p53 and DCC genes are deleted in more than 70 percent of the carcinomas. Figure 5.1 illustrates the theoretical steps involved in the progression from normal cells lining the colon to cancer cells.

TABLE 5.2 *Conceptual Models for Multistep Carcinogenesis*

Retinoblastoma	Two steps: loss of both alleles of the Rb tumor-suppressor gene on chromosome 13. Tumor usually appears by three years of age. Osteosarcomas may have similar mechanism.
Wilms' tumor	Two steps: loss of both alleles of the Wilms' tumor, tumor-suppressor gene on chromosome 11. Tumor usually appears in infants or young children. Rhabdomyosarcomas and hepatoblastomas of children may have similar mechanisms.
Burkitt's lymphoma	Two or more steps: infections with Epstein-Barr virus and malarial parasite allow active proliferation of B-cells. Such proliferation increases possibility for translocation of c-*myc* oncogene near immunoglobulin enhancer, thereby increasing the oncogene's expression. Tumor usually appears in early childhood in African children.
Cancer of the cervix	Four or more steps: infection with human papillomaviruses types 16 or 18. Activation of c-*neu* (or c-*erb*B) protooncogene. Carcinogens in cigarette smoke possibly induce changes in tumor-suppressor genes on chromosomes 3, 11, and 17 (p53 gene).
Cancer of the lung	Five or more steps: two protooncogenes, c-*myc* and c-K-*ras*, amplified; tumor-suppressor genes deleted from chromosomes 3 and 17. Tumor usually appears in older people. Cigarette smoke possibly involved in two steps.
Cancer of the colon	At least four to six steps: activation of protooncogenes c-K-*ras* and c-*myc* and inactivation of multiple tumor-suppressor genes on chromosomes 5 (APC gene), 17 (p53 gene), and 18 (DCC gene).

FIGURE 5.1 Progression to Colon Cancer

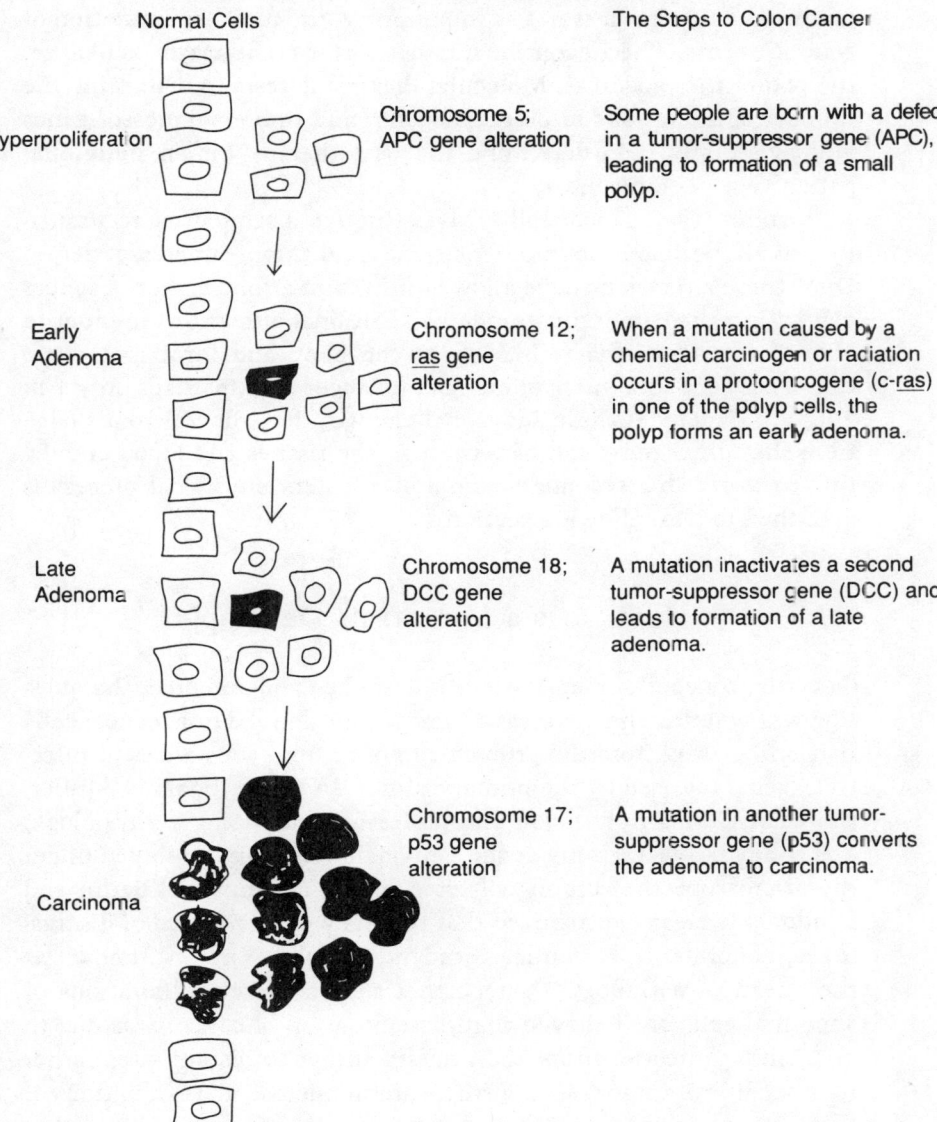

Normal Cells

The Steps to Colon Cancer

Poly/Hyperproliferation

**Chromosome 5;
APC gene alteration**

Some people are born with a defect in a tumor-suppressor gene (APC), leading to formation of a small polyp.

Early Adenoma

**Chromosome 12;
ras gene alteration**

When a mutation caused by a chemical carcinogen or radiation occurs in a protooncogene (c-_ras_) in one of the polyp cells, the polyp forms an early adenoma.

Late Adenoma

**Chromosome 18;
DCC gene alteration**

A mutation inactivates a second tumor-suppressor gene (DCC) and leads to formation of a late adenoma.

Carcinoma

**Chromosome 17;
p53 gene alteration**

A mutation in another tumor-suppressor gene (p53) converts the adenoma to carcinoma.

In some patients an alteration in chromosome 5 seems to promote the early hyperproliferation of normal colon epithelium. Also the activation of the _ras_ gene often occurs relatively early in adenomas during the accumulation of genetic alterations. In some other colon cancers it is a later event. Thus, although the progression of events tends to be regular, it is not as important as the total accumulation of genetic events. The greater the number of steps that have taken place, the poorer the prognosis. Molecular diagnostic tests to determine the number of alterations in protooncogenes and tumor-suppressor genes will eventually help determine the best therapy for an individual patient with colon cancer.

In summary, a cancer cell evolves through a sequential accumulation of alterations in its protooncogenes and tumor-suppressor genes. Once these alterations have allowed it to form a solid tumor, a cancer cell within the tumor must undergo additional alterations in order to allow it to disseminate throughout the body and form metastatic tumors. Of the total mass of malignant cancer cells, perhaps only 1 in 100,000 undergoes these additional changes that allow it to dislodge from the tumor mass and pass through the tissues and blood circulation to establish a secondary tumor at a distant site. That process is described in the following section.

How Does a Metastasis Develop?

Once the concept of metastasis was described and accepted, the question was whether the metastatic tumors were derived from cancer cells that broke away from the primary tumor or from substances or infective agents released by the primary tumor. In 1836, Johannes Müller, the great German physician and professor of pathology, physiology, and comparative anatomy at the University of Berlin, observed under the microscope the tumors collected in the museums in Berlin and London. He clearly recognized that tumors were composed of disorganized, abnormal cells. Müller's student, Rudolph Virchow, known as the "dean of pathology," agreed that tumors were proliferations of abnormal cells but believed that dissemination of cancer was due to noncellular infection from the primary tumor to distant sites rather than seeding of tumor cells. Further careful microscopic evaluations of the primary and metastatic tumors by pathologists eventually ruled in favor of the cellular origin of metastasis. Metastasis is now defined as the spread of cells from a primary tumor and their growth at new sites.

Early on it was believed that all cancers and all cells within every cancer were able to metastasize. Again, careful studies have indicated that this is not the case. Not all cancers metastasize, and only some of the cells within a cancer are capable of establishing a metastatic tumor. Although originally derived from a single cell, after many cell divisions the cancer cells present in both primary and metastatic tumors are now known to be heterogeneous, differing in a wide range of genetic and biological properties, including chromosome complements, enzymes, cell morphology, growth properties, and ability to invade adjacent tissues and produce metastases. In fact, only a few cells in a primary tumor have developed the genetic alterations that allow them to give rise to metastases. They must break off from the original tumor, enter the lymphatic or blood channels, and survive collisions with other cells and vessel walls. After eventually lodging in a small vessel, they must start to grow and invade through the vessel wall into the tissues of a new organ. There they must induce the growth of blood vessels *(angiogenesis)* to support the growth of their metastatic cell colony. Those circulating tumor cells that fail to complete any of the steps in the metastatic process are eliminated (see figure 5.2). It is easy to see why only a few cells in a primary tumor give rise to a metastasis.

What, exactly, is the metastatic process or cascade, as it has been called? Cancer research scientists who study metastasis usually begin with the origins of the cancer itself and proceed to the series of interrelated events in metastasis, as described here:

TUMOR INITIATION	Oncogene activation and tumor-suppressor gene inactivation.
TUMOR PROMOTION AND PROGRESSION	Additional oncogene and tumor-suppressor gene alterations, chromosome rearrangements, hormonal factors.
UNCONTROLLED PROLIFERATION	Progressive growth of cancer cells.
ANGIOGENESIS	The cancer cells secrete angiogenic factors, which stimulate the formation of capillaries from the surrounding tissues into the cancer.
INVASION	Normal tissues are separated from each other by intracellular stroma, also called matrix, and/or a defined basement membrane. To invade local tissues, tumor cells must pass through these barriers in a three-step process.
	The first step is tumor cell

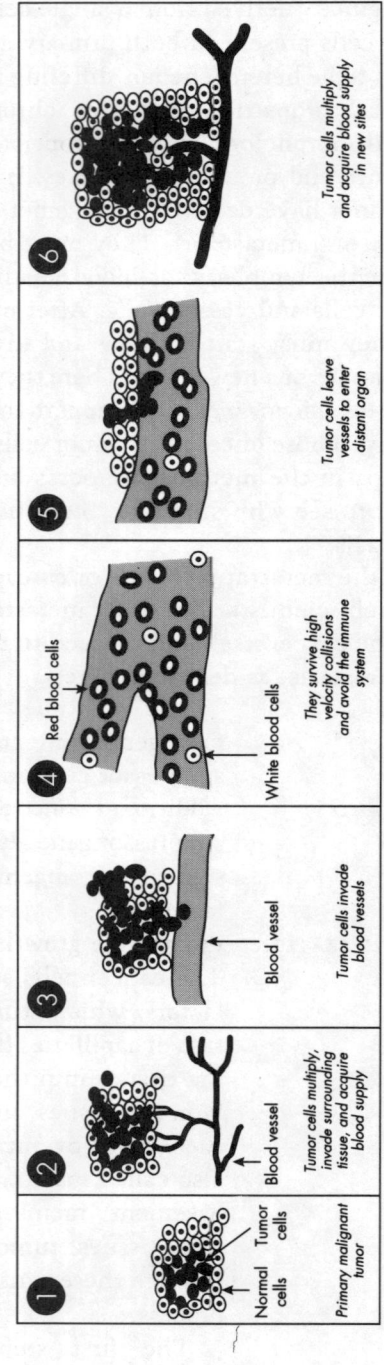

FIGURE 5.2   The Multistep Process of Metastasis

1
Normal cells
Tumor cells
Primary malignant tumor

2
Blood vessel
Tumor cells multiply, invade surrounding tissue, and acquire blood supply

3
Blood vessel
Tumor cells invade blood vessels

4
Red blood cells
White blood cells
They survive high velocity collisions and avoid the immune system

5
Tumor cells leave vessels to enter distant organ

6
Tumor cells multiply and acquire blood supply in new sites

Cancer cells have to be able to perform every step in the sequence in order to spread.

Reprinted with permission from Dawn Darling and David Tarin, "The Spread of Cancer in the Human Body," *New Scientist*, 1990: 52.

adherence, or attachment, to the proteins in the stroma or basement membrane. Following attachment, the tumor cells secrete enzymes that can locally degrade or dissolve the attachment glycoproteins and the proteins in the basement membranes. Several types of protein-dissolving enzymes, called proteases, have now been detected in tumor cells. These proteases are there in large enough amounts to overcome the natural protease inhibitors that are always present in the serum and stroma itself to protect the integrity of the membrane structures. Indeed, the outcome of the metastatic process depends on the balance between the proteases and their inhibitors or metastatic-suppressor proteins.

The tumor cell proteases include members of three major categories of proteases: serine proteases, cysteine proteases (both named for their sites of action on specific amino acids within the protein molecule), and metalloproteinases, named for their content of metal ions.

The third step in the invasion process is the migration of the tumor cell through the vascular wall into the circulation. The movement of tumor cells through the stroma and basement membrane mediated by the protein-dissolving enzymes is probably directed by chemical motility factors elaborated from both the host tissues and the tumor cells themselves.

DETACHMENT

Individual cancer cells or small

ARREST

MIGRATION

PROLIFERATION

SECONDARY METASTASIS

clumps of cancer cells are shed from the primary cancer into the circulation.

Cancer cells that survive mechanical stresses of circulation through lymph channels, veins, and arteries are stopped in small capillaries of various organs.

There the cancer cells grow and, perhaps by the same mechanisms as for initial invasion, burst through the vessel walls into the surrounding tissues of a new site.

The cancer cells in the new organ multiply, induce the growth of local capillaries, and respond to factors, specific for each organ, that influence their growth. The metastatic tumor can grow very large, sometimes larger than the primary tumor.

Following this series of events, the cells of the metastatic cancer can again invade the adjacent tissue, penetrate blood vessels, and reenter the circulation to form secondary metastases, or metastases of metastases.

In addition, clinical observations have suggested that certain tumors produce metastases only in specific organs. A hundred years ago Stephen Paget questioned whether the distribution of metastases from specific cancers to all organs was random. He reviewed the autopsy records of 735 women with breast cancer and discovered that metastases frequently occurred in lungs, liver, and bones but rarely in other organs. Subsequent studies confirmed Paget's findings about breast cancer and described specific patterns of spread for other cancers. Based on his observations, Paget theorized that the metastatic process was not random but predestined, in that the primary cancer released certain tumor cells, called "seeds," that had a special ability to grow in certain organs, or "soil." Metastatic tumors developed only when the "seed" cells matched the organ "soil."

At first it was suggested that the cancer cells dislodged from the primary tumor would enter the lymph or vein blood vessel, flow with the lymph or blood, and form metastases in the first organ that trapped them in its small capillaries. This does happen. Cancer cells entering veins are transported to the heart and then pumped in the arterial blood to the lungs, a common site of metastasis. But many other cancers metastasize to organs such as the liver and brain, instead of the lungs, and cannot be explained by the anatomy of the blood flow from tumors in various parts of the body to the lungs. Those seed cells must have passed through the lung capillaries and been distributed to organs that provided more receptive "soil."

Experimental studies of animals injected with cancer cells labeled with radioactive compounds or fluorescent dyes have shown that the cells do not all localize in the lungs but, in fact, reach every organ within about fifteen minutes (Fidler 1990). Metastases did form most often in the lungs, though, apparently because that "soil" was more suitable than the "soil" in the brain, liver, kidney, or muscle. Labeled cells were also detected in these other organs but did not grow into secondary tumors.

Clinical studies in human cancer patients have also been informative. When millions of cancer cells accumulate in the abdominal cavity of patients with certain types of cancer, one therapy involves artificially shunting these cells into the jugular vein. This procedure surprisingly did not increase the risk of metastasis, even though the cancer cells were coursing through the circulation. The most remarkable finding was in patients who already had metastases in certain organs before the shunt was inserted. In these cases, the number of metastatic tumors in the initially affected organ increased, but other organs remained free of metastases. These results support Paget's hypothesis that only a rare cancer cell among the millions of "seeds" is capable of forming a metastatic colony, and that this cell cannot grow indiscriminately in any organ but only in the "soil" of the target organ that is supportive of its growth.

What are the requirements or properties that might explain this selective process? Isaiah Fidler, who has devoted his entire scientific career to elucidating the mysteries of metastasis, lists as required factors for the successful metastatic cell—what he calls the decathlon champion—certain growth factors and angiogenic factors that stimulate capillary formation in the tumor. For the host "soil" to provide a favorable environment in a particular organ, it, too, must possess certain hormones and growth-promoting factors of its own. Determining the structure and the role of these substances will help lead to ways of interfering with and inhibiting the metastatic process.

It has also been suggested that oncogenes may be involved in the selection of more aggressive tumor cells with the capacity to metastasize. This idea is supported by the fact that in certain types of cancer, oncogene overexpression or amplification does correlate with the likelihood of metastatic activity. The amplification of erbB, an oncogene involved in breast cancer, has been detected in about 30 percent of breast cancer patients and is associated with an increase in the incidence of metastasis to axillary lymph nodes. When such amplification is found, more aggressive intervention seems warranted. Another example of oncogene amplification is found in the most malignant stages of neuroblastoma, involving extensive metastases. Here the N-myc oncogene has been overexpressed and produces an excess of its protein product.

What other factors play a role in the metastatic process? Only a few years ago, Patricia Steeg and Lance Liotta, scientists at the National Cancer Institute, discovered a gene with the ability to suppress the metastasis of cancer cells. First found in mouse melanoma cells, this metastatic-suppressor gene turned out to resemble closely other genes that are known to control developmental changes in simpler organisms. This provided the investigators with a clue that may allow them to determine the exact mechanism of the inhibition exhibited by the gene or its protein product. This new gene has been designated nm-23 (so called because it is non-metastatic and was the twenty-third gene tested from melanoma cells) and was found to be located on chromosome 17. One allele of the nm-23 gene has been shown to be deleted from the DNA of patients suffering from certain types of breast, kidney, colon/rectal, and lung cancers before those cancer cells metastasize. This suggests that such a loss increases the likelihood that these cells may spread to distant sites. Furthermore, both nm-23 alleles were found to be deleted from the cells of the lymph node metastases in a colon/rectal cancer patient. The fact that both alleles of the nm-23 gene are missing in metastatic cells provides supportive evidence that nm-23 is indeed involved in the suppression of metastasis.

Drawing our attention now to the protein product of the nm-23 gene, we find that it has been detected in breast and colon cancer cells. More to the point, preliminary findings indicate that the nm-23 protein activity increases in the primary cancer cells (before metastasis) but decreases as the cancers become metastatic. Again we have supportive evidence, this time pointing to the suppressor effect of the nm-23 protein product: When its activity diminishes or is lost, cancer cells are able to metastasize. Any alteration in the nm-23 gene or its protein product, it has been reasoned, could enhance the metastatic process. The hope is to apply this information in a clinical setting: A determination of the activity of the nm-23 protein in the cells of a given cancer patient might lead to an estimation of the likelihood of the metastatic spread of the disease. If the level is low, it might signal the need to intervene earlier with more drastic treatment.

Since metastasis is the most life-threatening phase of the cancer process, the quest for agents, including pharmaceuticals, that can interfere with this process is an urgent one. The more we understand about the structure and mechanism of action of a particular gene or its protein product in cancer, the better able we will be to intervene in the process. Steeg and Liotta believe that the protein for which the nm-23 gene encodes may be a key regulatory enzyme in a major signal transmission pathway that sends signals from many growth factors and hormones into the nucleus of the cell. There, the DNA is stimulated in some specific way and the signal is converted into a cellular response. This class of regulatory enzymes, which includes the nm-23 proteins, is called nucleoside diphosphate (NDP) kinases and plays a role in the ability of the cell to form a mitotic spindle, a process essential for orderly cell division. It is very encouraging to scientists to be able to find factors that control such fundamental processes in the cell, because cancer is a disease that results from disorderly cell division.

New Strategies to Combat Metastasis

Because we now view the cancer cell that is capable of metastasizing as different in its genetic makeup and protein (enzyme) products from both normal cells and primary cancer cells, it should, at least theoretically, be possible to target these cells selectively for earlier diagnostic strategies, prognostic evaluations, and treatment approaches. Any of the steps in the metastatic process we have outlined could, in principle, be blocked by appropriate therapeutic agents more specific than the standard treatments now in use.

As an example, let us examine one of the tumor cell proteases that is part of the invasion phase of metastasis, those called metalloproteinases. The gene that codes for a *tissue inhibitor* of these *metalloprotei-*

nases has been cloned, making possible the production of significant amounts of the protein product (TIMP) by recombinant DNA techniques, now called r-TIMP. This r-TIMP binds to and inhibits collagenase, a protein-dissolving enzyme closely associated with tumor cell invasion of metastatic sites. Not only does r-TIMP inhibit metastasis but it may also inhibit angiogenesis, the formation of new blood vessels in the developing metastatic tumor and essential for its growth. There are now tentative plans to use r-TIMP in patients with breast or prostate cancer who have developed metastases.

More clinical trials are planned for antimetastatic agents designed to block the spread of cancer cells and inhibit the growth of additional tumors. The specificity of these agents holds out great promise because their toxicity for normal cells may be lower, making their potential value immense.

PART II

THE CANCER PATIENT

Introduction

DURING THE YEARS SINCE THE NATIONAL CANCER ACT WENT INTO effect in 1971, not only have numerous breakthroughs about the causes of cancer been made in the laboratory but also much has been learned about better ways to diagnose cancer, to treat it more effectively and with fewer side effects, to manage it so that patients who cannot be cured can live longer and better lives, and in some cases to bring about long-term remissions (disease-free interludes after which the cancer sometimes recurs).

Back in 1971, the major types of cancer therapy—surgery, radiation, and chemotherapy—although sometimes curative, were somewhat limited. Chemotherapy, for example, was confined to a few effective but often toxic agents. Today numerous highly effective and less toxic drugs are available, and new ones, such as taxol, have been discovered. Additionally, many new surgical and X-ray treatments are in use. Cancer therapists now know much more about when to use combination therapies—that is, surgery, X ray, and/or chemotherapy as opposed to surgery or chemotherapy alone. And mammography has become a much safer and more accurate procedure since better pictures can be obtained with lower doses of X ray.

There has been a concerted effort since 1971, largely through the National Cancer Institute (NCI), to make sure that the latest advances in diagnosis and treatment get out to frontline physicians and the general public as quickly as possible. Detailed programs have been established at the National Cancer Institute for the diagnosis and treatment of every cancer, specific not only for the type of cancer but also for its extent or spread and the type of cell it involves. These treatment programs or protocols have been created, after years of studies sponsored by the NCI, to establish universal standards for treatment. Part II includes a discussion of how anyone—patient, family, or physician—can find out about these protocols.

Since 1971, the number of Cancer Centers in the United States has increased from three to fifty-seven. These centers bring together clinicians and research scientists to exchange information about the newest specialized treatments for cancer patients and promote public education about cancer. (See the appendix for a listing of these centers.) In order to be designated a Cancer Center, a hospital must meet certain rigid criteria involving cancer treatment, research activities, and community educational programs and must be supported by the National Cancer Institute. Programs are also in place to allow community hospitals to collaborate with Cancer Centers, so that patients who cannot be treated at major centers and their doctors can still get the best, most up-to-date information about diagnosis and treatment.

Chapter 6 describes the latest principles and strategies of cancer diagnosis, incorporating the changes that have been made as a result of the advances in understanding the molecular biology of cancer. Blood-test screening of older men, for example, should lead to earlier diagnosis and treatment of prostate cancer, so common in this group. Progress has also been made in evaluating the prognosis of breast cancer patients by measuring the level of a particular gene product in the cancer tissue. Women with high levels of this gene product are less likely to remain in remission after standard chemotherapy and are generally advised to undergo more aggressive treatment.

In chapter 7, we discuss the current status of cancer treatment. Improvements in treatment since 1971 have been due mainly to refinements in the standard surgical techniques, radiation, and chemotherapies. Women with breast cancer can now often be treated without the mutilating surgery of breast removal. Men with testicular cancer or prostate cancer can often not only be cured but assured of retaining sexual function. Some patients with laryngeal cancer can retain their voices, and those with bone cancer can retain their limbs. The most dramatic improvements have been achieved in childhood cancer, where two-thirds of all patients now survive at least five years.

Chapter 8 explains how to find out about clinical trials—experimental research programs—and what it is like to participate in them. A clinical protocol is reproduced in full, including patient eligibility, treatment plan, and complete clinical report.

Chapter 6

Diagnosis

THE WOMAN WITH A LUMP IN HER BREAST AND THE MAN WITH AN increasingly serious chronic cough should see their doctors. How would a doctor tackle these symptoms and attempt to determine whether breast cancer or lung cancer should be diagnosed? This chapter is a brief answer to that question.

The first responsibility lies with the individual, who should be aware of the American Cancer Society's seven basic warning signs and symptoms of cancer, any of which should prompt a visit to the doctor:

- Unusual bleeding or discharge
- A lump that does not go away
- A sore that does not heal within two weeks
- A change in bowel or bladder habits
- Persistent hoarseness or cough
- Indigestion or difficulty in swallowing
- Changes in a wart or mole.

The physician seeing a patient with any of these symptoms will devise a "diagnostic workup" to determine whether any of the major forms of cancer are present:

CARCINOMA   Most common cancer that develops in epithelial tissues, those that cover or line the cavities of the body—for example, skin, lung, bowel, kidney, breast, ovary, uterus, prostate.

SARCOMA	Cancer that develops in connective tissues, those that support or connect or surround other tissues and organs—for example, bone, cartilage, muscle.
LEUKEMIA	Cancer that develops in blood cells or blood-forming tissues—bone marrow and spleen.
LYMPHOMA	Cancer that develops in cells of lymph nodes.
MYELOMA	Cancer that develops in antibody-forming blood cells, plasma cells, and in bone marrow of pelvis, spine, ribs, and skull.
GERM CELL TUMOR	Cancer that develops in ovaries or testes.

The diagnostic procedures will vary somewhat according to the type and location of the suspected cancer. In part III we discuss the diagnostic strategies for the ten most common cancers in the United States.

The standard diagnostic workup for someone who is in the doctor's office because of a fear of having cancer will begin with a clinical history—the patient's description of his or her chief complaints and symptoms. This is also the time for the doctor to review previous illnesses, any exposures to tobacco or other carcinogens, and the occurrence of cancer or other major diseases in family members. A complete physical examination will then be made, including a rectal examination and examination of the prostate gland in men and breasts in women. Complete blood cell counts and hemoglobin level as well as urine analysis and a chest X ray will also be obtained.

If cancer is suspected after the doctor has determined the chief complaints, obtained a health history, and performed a complete physical examination, additional tests will be run to distinguish the type of cancer and to find out whether it has spread. Usually the most important single test for establishing a diagnosis of cancer is a biopsy.

In a biopsy, a piece of tissue is removed so that it can be examined under a microscope and found to be normal, benign, or cancerous. There are different kinds of biopsy techniques. *Incisional* biopsies cut out ("incise") only a piece of the tumor. *Excisional*, or total, biopsy removes the entire lump or tumor. *Needle aspiration* or *punch biopsies* use a needle or an instrument similar to a hole punch to extract tissue or fluid from a tumor mass. Many biopsies can be performed in the doctor's office. When a biopsy is performed in the operating room, the tissue may be examined by a quick method called "frozen section," in which thin slices or sections of the tissue are frozen, stained, and examined under the microscope. The pathologist's report to the surgeon waiting in the operating room may influence the immediate surgical attack on the tumor. Besides the frozen section, a "permanent section" is prepared on all biopsies by a multistage procedure that yields stained, thin slices of the biopsied tissue prepared for precise microscopic diagnosis. It takes several days to get the results of a permanent section.

The pathologist examines the biopsy for microscopic characteristics of cancer tissue or cells. These characteristics consist mainly of evidence of disruption of normal tissue architecture by the invasion of sheets of cells with bizarre shapes and sizes and with abnormal, swollen nuclei. Many of the cells with malignant forms are replicating via mitotic division with unusual chromosome numbers and alignments. The actively dividing cells with bizarre mitotic figures often stain more deeply than the normal cells, thus giving malignant tissue a grossly overstained appearance under the microscope.

Sometimes the diagnostic workup will uncover findings that suggest the patient has leukemia. These clinical and laboratory findings might include bleeding from various sites (such as the mouth), easy bruising, paleness, alterations in white blood cell counts (*leukemia* means "white blood" and is sometimes caused by the large numbers of white blood cells in patients with this disease), anemia, and decreased platelet counts. To aid in the diagnosis of leukemia, a specimen of bone marrow is extracted through a needle inserted into the hip bone or sternum. The pathologist examines this specimen microscopically for changes in the normal cells and for the presence of various types of leukemic cells, which are altered forms of normal red or white blood cells.

The final pathology report of the biopsy or bone marrow examination is crucial not only for the diagnosis of the type and malignant characterization of the cancer but also because it is the basis on which all future decisions will be made. What type of treatment will be most effective? What is the patient's immediate and lifelong prognosis?

Besides the biopsy and bone marrow examinations, a complete diagnostic workup for cancer sometimes requires a number of other tests, among them additional X-ray examinations, computerized tomography (CT scan), magnetic resonance imaging (MRI), ultrasound, radionuclide scans, and endoscopy. Brief descriptions of these tests follow:

ADDITIONAL X RAYS

Besides routine chest X rays, other kinds of X rays are useful in identifying cancers of the breast and gastrointestinal tract and in detecting metastatic cancers in the lung, brain, bone, and liver. In addition to these standard (plain film) X-ray examinations, many others use a contrast medium to help outline the organ being X-rayed (contrast film). For instance, a barium enema X-ray examination is a contrast film in which a solution containing barium is introduced as an enema to outline the colon and rectum. Many other contrast films using various radiopaque substances can be used to diagnose cancers of the brain, bronchi, gallbladder, bladder, kidney, female genital tract, and lymph nodes. These are named after the organ being examined; for instance, cholecystogram for gallbladder, lymphangiogram for lymph nodes, and angiogram for blood vessels.

CT SCANS
(COMPUTERIZED
TOMOGRAPHY SCANS)

These are a series of X-ray examinations that zero in on small slices of tissue throughout the body. The X-ray images from these slices are read, or "scanned," by a computer on the basis of light or dark shadows, which indicate the density of the tissues in the slice. By reading the computer analysis of the X-ray pictures of each slice, the radiologist can reconstruct the structures, including normal or cancer tissues, in any segment of the body—for instance, the head, chest, or abdomen.

MRI (MAGNETIC
RESONANCE IMAGING)

This technique uses magnets rather than X-ray tubes to obtain pictures of slices or cross-sections of the body, much as CT scans. It relies upon the radio signals emitted in various tissues of the body when a patient is placed in a high magnetic field. The great advantages of MRI are that it shows exquisite anatomical detail of structure and provides physiological tissue information, revealing otherwise invisible structures such as cartilage, muscles, tendons, and vascular flow. MRI studies show normal tissues as well as abnormal tissues, benign as well as malignant. The images tend to be sharper and more detailed than CT scan pictures and are especially useful for detecting tumors in the brain and liver. On the other hand, MRI scans are not better than mammograms in detecting breast tumors. MRI is expected to evaluate responsiveness of the tumor during the course of therapy and to indicate the recurrence of a tumor. In general, patients tolerate the MRI procedure well, but because they must be placed in an enclosed tunnel, claustrophobia can be a problem. Also, patients with metallic implants such as pacemakers cannot be exposed to the magnetic field.

ULTRASOUND

In this technique, a probe sends out bursts of rapid sound waves called sonar or ultrasounds over the surface of the body. These waves are reflected by, or bounce off, the internal tissues, yielding a picture of the echoes on a screen. The echoes can then be photographed by an attached camera. As with CT scan pictures and MRI pictures, ultrasound pictures can detect tumor masses but, unlike MRI and CT scans, cannot distinguish between benign and malignant ones. Ultrasound is useful in detecting tumors of the uterus, ovaries, stomach, liver, pancreas, and kidneys. It is sometimes used to detect breast cancer but is not useful in diagnosing lung cancer.

RADIONUCLIDE SCANS

For these tests, also called nuclear scans, a minute amount of a radionuclide-tagged compound—such as radioactive iodine or gallium—is injected into a vein. After brief intervals, during which the compound can localize in various organs and tissues, a series of scans is obtained by a mobile scanner—a stationary camera that records the radioactive emissions on a film. The tissues or organs in which the radioactive compound has localized emit more radiation and are recorded as dark areas in the pictures. Such radioactive scans can not only diagnose cancer but also detect metastatic cancer when used as part of a metastatic workup.

ENDOSCOPY

A number of different tests are included under the term endoscopy, all using an optical instrument—a "scope"—to observe an interior part of the body. The scopes can be rigid tubes with a light on the end, or flexible plastic fibers (fiberoptics) that transmit light and contain a telescope on the end. The various scopes can not only observe but sometimes biopsy various organs such as bronchoscope (for bronchus), esophagoscope (for esophagus), and colonoscope (for colon).

In addition to these tests, and depending upon the type of cancer suspected, a series of blood tests can be done to detect "markers" in the blood for specific cancers. These tests as well as the biopsies, bone marrow examinations, CT scans, MRI, and other tests just mentioned will be discussed as they apply to each of the major types of cancer considered in part III. Finally, a series of new tests is under development. Some of these are based on detection of enhanced activity of oncogenes or loss of activity of tumor-suppressor genes as described in chapters 3 and 4.

There may seem to be a surprising number of different tests to establish the diagnosis of cancer, but it is crucial to ascertain the exact type of cancer, whether it is malignant, and whether it has spread. The entire treatment program that will be devised for the patient—as discussed in the next chapter—depends on the outcome of this wide spectrum of diagnostic tests.

Since the proper diagnosis and treatment of cancer are obviously of enormous importance, a common question is whether a second opinion should be sought. The answer is yes. Most physicians are completely understanding of this issue and will readily provide patients with the names of consulting pathologists and of physicians who will give a second opinion about the pathology findings and the proposed treatment. A patient's insurance company or health maintenance organization will also supply the names of consultants, as will the American Cancer Society and the Cancer Information Service (1-800-4-CANCER).

Chapter 7

Treatment

THE EARLIEST ATTEMPTS TO TREAT CANCER WERE DESCRIBED IN THE
Papyrus Ebers, an Egyptian document written about 1600 B.C.
These attempts consisted of surgery or the injection of mixtures of
ingredients such as fresh dates, limestone, and water into the tumor
mass. Thereafter, along with surgical excision of accessible cancers, a
wide variety of herbal and chemical concoctions were administered to
cancer patients. Some were salves that usually contained arsenic or
other metals that had a caustic effect on the superficial cancer and
surrounding tissues. By 1865, a German physician named Lissauer
reported two patients with leukemia who had a temporary (clinical)
response to arsenic-containing Fowler's solution. This treatment for
leukemia was used until the early 1900s, when radiation therapy and
the chemical benzol were tried with little success.

In 1893, William B. Coley, a New York surgeon, noted the regression of a sarcoma in a patient who also had erysipelas, a streptococcal
infection. He concocted a mixture of streptococci and another microorganism, Bacillus prodigious, that had objective effects in some patients with sarcomas. In 1898, he reported his mixed-toxin treatment
in the *Journal of the American Medical Association.* It proved to be
dangerous, with unpredictable effects. Research efforts to characterize
the active ingredient suggested that it was a polysaccharide (sugar
compound), but its use in cancer therapy remains undefined.

By 1880, surgery to remove internal cancers was the major method of cancer therapy, to be joined by radiation therapy in 1900
and chemotherapy in the 1940s. Recently a number of new treatments have come into use for certain cancers: immunotherapy with

tuberculosis antigens and tumor-cell antigens to stimulate the immune system; hyperthermia, which directs increased temperature at the cancer; photodynamic therapy, which uses a combination of chemical compounds that can be activated to kill cancer cells when they are exposed to light from a laser beam; and biological response modifiers such as interferons, interleukins, colony-stimulating factors, and tumor necrosis factors, natural biological substances (or their genetically engineered equivalents) that inhibit the growth of cancer cells.

On the current scene are an array of additional strategies to treat cancer by taking advantage of the new knowledge about the two classes of cancer genes (oncogenes and tumor-suppressor genes) as well as genes involved with metastasis. These theoretical treatments will be described in more detail in the next chapter. First we will discuss the most common treatments for cancer today: surgical therapy, radiation therapy, and chemotherapy.

Surgical Therapy

During the Renaissance and into the seventeenth century, surgeons began to do extensive operations. A French barber/surgeon, Ambroise Paré (1510–90), rose to become surgeon to four French kings. (Barbers often performed surgical operations during that era.) His skillful and conservative approach to cancer surgery is illustrated by his description of a patient with a cancer of the lip:

> Sometimes one may otherwise and more happily cure cancers of the lip without applying caustics or any similar thing. . . . The way is this: Pass a threaded needle through the cancer so the thread held in the left hand can lift and control the cancer without any of its escaping. One can then cut to good flesh with scissors in the right hand; and cut so that a layer of good flesh of the lip remains to serve as a base and foundation for regeneration of flesh in place of the portion amputated, supposing the cancer has not taken root and spread from top to bottom. This done, having let enough blood flow from within and without, at the right and left of the amputation, make deep enough incisions with the razor so that later, when one would draw together and unite the edges of the wound . . . the flesh would be more obedient to the thread and needle.
> [In Shimkin 1977]

The father of German surgery, Wilhelm Fabry (1560–1624), was a daring and inventive surgeon who described his vast surgical experience in twenty books, most of which were collected in his *Opera*, published in 1646. He devised the tourniquet to control bleeding. He also developed a special forceps for amputating a breast with cancer; the instrument constricted the base of the breast while a blade swept the organ off the chest wall. He described a number of operations for breast cancer that included excision of enlarged lymph nodes.

The modern era of surgery for internal organs began in the United States in 1809, when Ephram MacDowell successfully excised a large ovarian tumor from a Mrs. Jane Crawford. This and thirteen subsequent ovarian excisions by MacDowell stimulated other surgeons to conduct elective abdominal surgery. In 1846, two dentists, William Morton and Crawford Long, administered ether to anesthetize a patient undergoing surgical excision of a submaxillary gland and a segment of the tongue. In 1867, following up on Louis Pasteur's observations that carbolic acid inhibited bacterial growth, Joseph Lister spearheaded its use to reduce bacterial infections associated with surgery.

These two milestones—the use of anesthesia to reduce the pain of surgery and the use of antiseptic techniques to reduce infection following surgery—led to the greatly increased use of surgical therapy for tumors. From the 1860s through the mid-1940s, numerous highly complex surgical techniques were devised by cancer surgeons to remove cancers and even pulmonary, liver, and brain metastases.

While many new surgical techniques have allowed for the successful resections of more and more cancers, the development of other treatment strategies such as preoperative radiation or chemotherapy have allowed surgeons to reduce the extent of surgical procedures required for some cancers. Technical innovations continue to improve the surgeon's ability to treat cancer. These include microsurgical techniques to suture together tiny blood vessels, useful in making grafts for reconstruction, and the development of fiberoptic endoscopic equipment that allows for biopsy of various internal lesions without resorting to large incisions. But for many cancers, surgery alone to remove a solid tumor that is localized at one site is still the best treatment and offers an excellent chance for cure.

In *specific* surgery, besides excising the discrete visible tumor, the surgeon will also excise some of the adjacent normal-appearing tissue to ensure removal of any cancer cells that might not be visible but that might have spread from the main tumor mass and could possibly cause a recurrence. The pathologist who examines the excised cancer and adjacent tissue microscopically can confirm whether the entire cancer was removed or whether cancer cells had invaded the adjacent tissues. *Radical* surgery consists of the removal not only of the cancer and adjacent tissues but also of the nearby organs and lymph nodes that might have been invaded by cancer cells.

While both specific and radical types of surgery are meant to be, and often are, curative, another surgical technique called *palliative* surgery is used not in an effort to cure but, rather, to treat the complications of the cancer, such as pain, recurrent tumors, or metastasis, and thus to offer the cancer patient a more comfortable life. Palliative surgery is also used to remove hormone-secreting glands, such as the ovaries or testes, which stimulate growth of some breast or prostate cancer. Excision of such glands has a palliative effect on these cancers.

Less common types of surgery employ the coagulating effect of electric current *(electrosurgery)*, freezing applications of liquid nitrogen *(cryosurgery)*, and directed laser beams *(laser surgery)*. Each of these techniques has been found to be useful for specific types of cancer: electrosurgery has been used successfully to treat cancers of the skin and rectum; cryosurgery for cancers of the skin, head, and neck; and laser surgery for selected cancers of the larynx, esophagus, and lung.

Before any surgery is performed, it is important that all the appropriate diagnostic tests have been completed (as described in the previous chapter) so that a comprehensive plan of treatment based on the stage of the cancer can be established in advance. Besides the routine diagnostic tests, and in view of the current concern about contamination with the AIDS virus by any blood that may be required for transfusion to replace blood lost at the time of surgery, it is important to consider storing an appropriate amount (one or more pints) of the patient's own blood prior to surgery. This has become a common practice when the patient's health and blood supply allow.

Any of the types of surgery should be performed by surgeons specializing in cancer surgery, who have three or more years of advanced training and Board Certification in surgical techniques in either general surgery or subspecialties, such as gynecology for cancers of the female genital tract, thoracic surgery for cancers of the chest, urology for cancers of the kidney, bladder, prostate, and male sex organs, or neurosurgery for brain cancers.

A cancer surgeon should be chosen by obtaining the names of highly qualified candidates from your primary physician or from the local Medical Association. It is also important, and often an insurance company requirement, to obtain a second opinion from another surgeon. The surgery should be conducted in a hospital with a cancer program approved by the American College of Surgeons or in a Cancer Center affiliated with a medical school. Such hospitals will have not only qualified cancer surgeons but also anesthesiologists who are also highly trained and certified by the American Board of Anesthesiology. The selection of such doctors and hospitals will reduce the risks associated with any surgery or anesthesia.

Radiation Therapy

X rays were discovered by Wilhelm Conrad Roentgen, a German professor of physics. In 1895, he published a paper, "On a New Kind of Ray"—which he named X ray—that was a landmark in science and medicine. Radiation as a scientific discipline was an immediate sensation, and Roentgen received the first Nobel Prize in physics in 1901.

Others noted that fluorescence was involved in the formation of X rays and looked at various naturally fluorescent substances as possible sources of X rays. In 1896, Antoine Henri Becquerel, a French scientist, found that uranium ore darkened photographic plates. It was concluded that the radiation given off by uranium was similar to X rays.

Marie Sklodowska, a Polish student in physics at the Sorbonne in Paris, and Pierre Curie, whom she married, followed up on Becquerel's observations and discovered in pitchblende ore, containing uranium, a substance that contained two million times as much radiation as uranium. They separated the new substance and called it radium. The Nobel Prize in physics in 1903 was shared by Becquerel, Marie Curie, and Pierre Curie. Thereafter it was observed that X rays and radium could damage body tissues. Within a year after Roentgen's discovery, "caustic" applications of X-ray beams were used to treat cancer.

Electromagnetic radiation consists of gamma radiation and X rays. Gamma rays are produced by the decay of radioactive isotopes, such as cobalt, with added electrons. X rays, on the other hand, are produced by electrical machines. At present, various forms of radiation therapy are used to treat over 50 percent of all cancer patients; only surgery is a more frequent treatment. Different ranges, or voltages, of electromagnetic radiation are used in clinical practice. The lowest range is called superficial radiation, the medium range is called orthovoltage, and the highest, supervoltage. Two types of radiation techniques are used. One, brachytherapy, is given close to or within the target tissue or organ, and the other, teletherapy, which uses an orthovoltage or a supervoltage machine, is given several feet or more from the patient.

Radiation biologists, who study the effects of radiation on living cells, have discovered that radiation damages DNA. Large doses of radiation cause such extensive damage to the DNA that the cells are killed; however, cells exposed to smaller doses of radiation have mechanisms to repair the slightly damaged DNA, and the cells can survive. The doses of radiation used to treat cancer are carefully adjusted to kill cancer cells, which are often more sensitive to the radiation than the adjacent normal cells. With each radiation treatment cancer cells are killed, and as they disintegrate the tumor shrinks.

Two major types of radiation are used to treat cancer: external-beam radiation teletherapy and internal radiation. External-beam radiation teletherapy consists of the delivery of X rays, gamma rays, or neutrons by various machines, such as standard orthovoltage, super-voltage, cobalt machines, or linear accelerators. External-beam therapy delivered to tumors by these different types of apparatus is the most commonly used radiation therapy for many cancers.

After twenty to thirty years of increasing clinical uses of radiation therapy, it is now possible to use small, "fractionated" applications over prolonged courses and kill cancer cells while sparing adjacent normal cells. The ultimate goal of curative radiation therapy is to achieve a favorable "therapeutic index"—that is, to cause the cancer cells to be destroyed and eliminated from the tissues without causing serious damage to healthy cells nearby.

With internal radiation, radium or other radioactive material is placed directly into the tumor. Most commonly, small radium needles or seed implants are used. But other radioactive materials such as cesium, iodine, gold, phosphorus, or iridium may be inserted surgically into the tumor in sealed needles or metal tubes, or, if in liquid form, given orally or injected into the tumor. The implanted needles or tubes are removed after the specific calculated dose of irradiation has been delivered locally to the tumor. Internal radiation can be used in cancers of the mouth, tongue, thyroid, breast, vagina, brain, lung, and prostate.

Radiation therapy can be administered according to three strategies: (1) as the curative form of therapy; (2) in combination with surgery and/or chemotherapy; or (3) as a palliative treatment for advanced cancer. It should not be undertaken until the patient has had a complete diagnostic evaluation and has come to an agreement with the cancer specialists on a comprehensive plan for all forms of treatment. In addition to establishing a course of treatment, the diagnostic workup must assure that the patient's general state of health can withstand radiation therapy. The radiation therapist, an M.D. who is extensively trained and certified by the American Board of Radiology, will also make a series of preliminary evaluations to determine the specific dose and delivery of the form of radiation therapy to be used. He or she will conduct a series of procedures to localize the tumor precisely and to determine the exact aim of the treatment beam. Localization of the tumor requires standard radiography as well as ultrasonography and, especially, computerized tomography (CT). CT is especially useful in delineating normal tissue and tumor tissue. For specific localization of the treatment beam, a radiation simulator is used. This is a device that mimics the treatment machine by substituting superficial radiation for the treatment beams and producing radiographs that indicate where the treatment beams will hit.

Curative radiation therapy, used with no other forms of cancer therapy, is now possible for certain cancers of the skin, cervix, head and neck, and Hodgkin's disease. Modern equipment that can deliver external radiation, such as supervoltage machines, offers a great improvement over the original orthoradiation machines. The newer machines emit high doses of radiation that can be sharply focused deep into the body and can destroy cancer tissues with minimal "scatter" injury to surrounding normal tissues and organs.

Curative radiation therapy is clearly the treatment of choice when the accumulated cancer treatment experience of the specific cancers provides impressive evidence to support its use. Such evidence exists for radiation treatment of Hodgkin's disease and some other lymphomas, as well as cancers of the skin, prostate, bladder, head, and neck. Another reason to choose radiation therapy in an effort to cure a specific cancer is when the outcome with surgery looks no better than that with radiation but would be much harder on the patient in terms of loss of function or disfigurement.

The second use of radiation therapy is as an adjunctive therapy, in combination with surgery and/or chemotherapy. These other modalities may be the treatment of choice, but radiation therapy is used either to shrink the cancer before surgery or to kill residual cancer cells not removed by surgery, including those cancer cells that may have spread to adjacent lymph nodes to which the cancer drains. This is a common treatment for Hodgkin's disease and rectal cancer. Radiation is also sometimes combined with hyperthermia—

that is, heating of the cancer—in an effort to enhance its cell-killing action.

The third use of radiation therapy is for palliation of side effects of cancer, for example, shrinking tumors that are pressing on nerves and causing pain, or shrinking brain metastases that are causing nausea and vomiting. Additionally, tumors that are blocking the gastrointestinal tract or the airways to the lungs can be reduced in size by radiation therapy to restore function.

External-beam radiation therapy is usually given in the Radiation Therapy department of a hospital. It consists of a series of exposures to the beams, a few minutes for five days a week over the course of several weeks, sometimes longer. The treatments are completely painless, although some patients feel a sensation of warmth or tingling. Treatment schedules, of course, vary for different types of cancer.

All patients are understandably concerned about the side effects of the radiation therapy itself. According to the target areas of the therapy and individual responses, side effects vary widely from none to severe. One of the most common reactions to external-beam radiation is the feeling of lethargy or fatigue. This can be helped if the patient reduces his or her level of activity and gets more sleep. Other reactions might include skin changes, such as dryness, itching, and darkening, hair loss, and local reactions following radiation to head and neck, abdomen, or other areas of exposure. Some patients also experience nausea and vomiting after radiation therapy, which can often be controlled by any number of effective antinausea drugs given orally or rectally.

Chemotherapy

Chemotherapy is the administration of various chemical compounds—drugs—for the treatment of cancer. The term *chemotherapy* was coined by Paul Erhlich, the great German scientist who developed animal models of infectious diseases to test the usefulness of various substances (chemicals and antibiotics) as treatment for these diseases in animals. This strategy was applied to cancer in the early 1900s by George Clowes in the United States, who tested the usefulness of various chemicals in treating cancers that had been transplanted into animals.

Between 1906 and 1940, numerous published reports described success in inhibiting such transplanted tumors in rodents. The substances tested for antitumor activity included salts of heavy metals, dyes, and various organic and biological products. A compilation by Helen Dyer in 1949 listed 5,031 substances tested for anticancer activity, most of which showed none.

Cancer chemotherapy came into general use long after surgical and radiation therapy and has proved to be remarkably helpful in treating leukemias, lymphomas, and certain solid tumors when used either alone or in combination with these other two standard therapies. The first useful chemotherapeutic agent for human cancer was a curious spinoff of the secret chemical warfare program used in both world wars. Seamen in World War II who were accidentally exposed to mustard gas following an explosion were observed to develop a depletion of their bone marrow and lymph cells. This observation led to the experimental use of nitrogen-mustard compounds, called alkylating agents, in patients with Hodgkin's disease and other lymphomas at Yale–New Haven Medical Center in 1943.

Work began at Yale under the cloak of wartime secrecy. The investigators, Drs. Alfred Gilman, Louis Goodman, and Frederick Philips, under contract with the Office of Scientific Research and Development, noted that nitrogen mustards were remarkably toxic to normal lymphoid tissue. Thomas Dougherty then tested a nitrogen mustard in a mouse with a transplanted lymphoma. The encouraging result led to a trial in humans. The first patient had an X-ray–resistant lymphosarcoma and was given a nitrogen mustard daily for ten days. The response was dramatic. More patients were treated successfully at Yale Medical Center, the University of Chicago, and Memorial Hospital in New York. The findings began to be published in 1946 when the secrecy restriction was lifted, but the full story was not told until 1963.

Even though the original nitrogen-mustard compound used intravenously was extremely toxic, causing severe nausea and vomiting in the recipients, it did show promise during the mid-1940s as a selective killer of rapidly growing cells, especially lymphoma cells. With these hopeful findings, other types of cell-killing compounds were aggressively sought between 1940 and 1975.

It was suspected that many chemicals would prove useful for the treatment of human cancer. From 1955 until 1975, the National Cancer Institute used an animal model, the mouse L1210 leukemia, to identify compounds that retard the progress of leukemia. By 1975, about 40,000 compounds had been tested using this model, including many of the currently available anticancer drugs active against human leukemias and lymphomas. Other screening systems were subsequently developed, including the use of cancer cells maintained in cultures *in vitro*. New chemotherapeutic agents are still being sought. Today the following tumors are sometimes curable by chemotherapy: acute lymphocytic leukemia in children and adults, Hodgkin's disease, Wilms' tumors, Burkitt's lymphoma, non-Hodgkin's lymphomas, acute myelogenous leukemia, trophoblastic tumors, ovarian cancer, testicular cancer, and rhabdomyosarcoma. Adjuvant chemotherapy (with surgery or radiation therapy) has successfully treated breast cancer, colon and rectal cancer, bone sarcoma, and soft-tissue sarcoma.

Following the initial discovery that nitrogen-mustard compounds showed temporary effectiveness in human leukemia, in 1948, Sidney Farber, at the Boston's Childrens Hospital, observed that an anti-metabolite (a compound that interferes with normal cellular metabolism of folic acid) called aminopterin prolonged the lives of leukemic children. The startlingly beneficial, albeit temporary, effectiveness of this drug in childhood leukemia helped launch more widespread use of chemotherapy in cancer. Thereafter a natural plant antibiotic, actinomycin-D, when used following surgery and radiation therapy, apparently cured children with Wilms' tumor.

During the 1970s, clinical trials (experimental research programs) of many types of cell-killing agents identified in screening tests were conducted. The agents included alkylating agents related to nitrogen mustard, other antimetabolites like aminopterin, other natural products from plants like actinomycin-D, and various hormones. In fact, clinical trials of these four classes of chemotherapeutic agents are still in progress, with the goal of identifying more effective, safer, less toxic compounds.

Taking clues from the treatment of childhood Wilms' tumor, in which the combination of surgery and radiation therapy had increased successful outcomes, and with actinomycin-D appearing to improve the outcome even more and lead to some cures, physicians in Cancer Centers began to use such combined therapy in adult cancers. Some adult cancers shrank in size dramatically after the administration of chemotherapeutic agents, but, disappointingly, they usually slowly grew back.

Then in the 1950s it was discovered that childhood tuberculosis could be successfully cured by the administration of a combination of compounds. A single agent such as streptomycin could cause a dramatic temporary improvement in the tuberculosis patient's condition, but after several months the patient would relapse. It was soon discovered that the combined use of several agents given for several months, followed by the continual use of one or more of them for a year or two, could cure the child's tuberculosis.

When the streptomycin alone was used, it killed most of the tuberculosis organisms. But some survived and were resistant to the killing effects of the drug; they could grow back and cause the relapse. The use of several drugs at the same time prevented the emergence of tuberculous organisms that were resistant, and thus all the organisms were killed and the patient was cured. This strategy was soon transposed to the treatment of childhood leukemia. As with tuberculosis, it was observed that the use of a single drug, aminopterin, could cause a dramatic temporary remission of this disease, only to be followed by a relapse. The leukemic cells, resistant to the killing effects of a single agent, would grow back. The use of several antileukemic agents, followed by a year of maintenance therapy with one or two of them, prolonged the life expectancy of leukemic children and cured many of them.

As its success was demonstrated more and more, chemotherapy came into general use by the 1970s. The National Cancer Institute now estimates that 15 percent of clinical cancers can be cured by chemotherapy alone, and about 50,000 cancer patients are cured annually through various combinations of surgery, radiation therapy, and chemotherapy. Combined therapy is now the most common way to treat cancer.

Chemotherapeutic agents can be administered orally, by intramuscular injections, or by intravenous injection. The agents can enter the bloodstream after being absorbed from the stomach or the muscle tissues, or directly (intravenously). In a few cancers, such as basal-cell carcinoma of the skin, they are also applied directly to the lesion, as an ointment. The blood evenly distributes the drugs to all parts of the body. An exception to this process is when the agent is injected through a catheter in a blood vessel leading directly to an organ, such as the liver. This is called *regional perfusion* of the agent. In this example, a liver tumor would receive a more concentrated dose of the agent than other tissues.

Cells, especially actively dividing cells, exposed to these different kinds of agents are killed by various mechanisms that usually act at different stages of the mitotic cycle. Alkylating agents are an exception. They do not act at a specific phase of the cell cycle, but rather bind nonspecifically to DNA and proteins to inhibit cell growth.

Antimetabolites are agents that often mimic and substitute for normal nucleic-acid building blocks that interfere with the synthesis of normal DNA, RNA, and proteins. One antimetabolite, 6-mercapto-purine, developed by George Hitchings at the Burroughs-Wellcome Company and tested clinically by Joseph Burchenal at the Memorial Cancer Hospital in New York, was found to be effective in childhood leukemia. Another antimetabolite, 5-Fluorouracil (5-FU), was invented and synthesized by Charles Heidelberger at the McArdle Laboratory for Cancer Research, at the University of Wisconsin. Tested clinically by the Wisconsin group, it proved useful in treating solid tumors, especially of the breast, colon, and rectum.

The natural-product type of chemotherapeutic agent consists of compounds, alkaloids, derived from plants such as the periwinkle or from antibiotics from molds. The agents are cell cycle–specific in their action—for instance, the mold antibiotic actinomycin-D is inserted between the bases of nucleic acids and stops cell division at the S, or DNA synthetic, stage. Fortunately, these agents kill cancer cells more than normal cells.

Hormonal manipulation can be used for cancer chemotherapy either by administering hormones, or their antagonists, to the patient, or by removing hormone-secreting organs such as the ovaries or testes from the patient.

George Thomas Beatson of Glasgow, Scotland, was the first surgeon to remove the ovaries of premenopausal women with advanced breast cancer. In 1896, he described the temporary regression of breast cancer following such surgery, thereby demonstrating the partial hormonal dependence of one human cancer. In performing such ovariectomy in breast cancer patients, he may have been acting on the advice of the German surgeon Albert Schingingers, who suggested such a procedure in 1889. Schingingers thought that the prognosis of breast cancer was better in older women and that younger women could be made "prematurely old by removing their ovaries" (Shimkin 1977, p. 178). But it was Beatson who actually conducted this innovative surgery for breast cancer. It remained the standard treatment until the 1930s, when it was replaced by the administration of hormones.

The usefulness of surgical removal of the testes in prostate cancer had its origins in the observation of J. W. White of Philadelphia that castration shrank the prostate glands of dogs. He also reported that castration had a beneficial effect on prostatic enlargement in man and published his findings in 1904. The procedure was abandoned, however, until 1941, when Charles Brenton Huggins at the University of

Chicago reported that patients with advanced cancer of the prostate gland showed a dramatic improvement after their testicles were removed. The procedure is also especially helpful in the alleviation of bone pain caused by metastases. Subsequent studies by Huggins revealed that injections of the synthetic female hormone estrogen, called diethylstilbestrol, caused the same regression of prostatic cancer as did castration. This ushered in the modern era of hormonal therapy for cancer. For discovering the hormonal control of prostatic cancer, Huggins was awarded the Nobel Prize in Physiology and Medicine in 1966.

A successor to Huggins at Chicago, Edward V. Jensen, reported that prostatic cancer responded to female sex hormones because of the presence of estrogen receptors within the cancer cells. The exact mechanism by which hormones act as therapeutic agents for certain cancers such as breast and prostate cancer is not completely understood, but they seem to be involved in regulation of growth-stimulating factors that enhance the growth of cancer cells.

The use of chemotherapeutic agents in cancer patients has been evolving since the 1950s. Thousands of potentially useful agents have been screened in cultures of cancer cells, in experimental animals, and eventually in patients with cancer. Large clinical trials of the agents have been conducted in many collaborating Cancer Centers under the auspices of the National Cancer Institute.

Clinical trials continue both in the United States and abroad, in the quest for even more effective agents. The optimal chemotherapy for specific cancers is determined by the results of these trials and is called a *protocol*. The protocol is the exact dose of the drug, the method of administration (oral or intravenous, for example), the interval between doses, and the length of treatment.

Physicians who direct chemotherapy treatments have had special training in the use of the various agents or combinations of agents. Usually they began their training in internal medicine, hematology, or pediatrics and, with additional training, then became medical or pediatric oncologists. The optimal care of an individual cancer patient is obtained through the coordination of the surgeon, radiation therapist, and medical or pediatric oncologist who prescribes the chemotherapy and often the general care of the patient.

The thought of receiving "chemo" is terrifying to many cancer patients. This public attitude is based in part on the early experience with chemotherapeutic agents such as nitrogen mustard, which caused such severe side effects as nausea, vomiting, hair loss, and burning pain at the site of the injection if the drug leaked out of the vein.

Fortunately, the type of drugs and methods of administration now used generally have fewer, less serious side effects or toxicity, but some do still cause severe reactions. Although some chemotherapeutic drugs, like standard drugs, intrinsically cause nausea and vomiting, it must be remembered that while anticancer drugs selectively kill cancer cells, they also kill some other rapidly dividing cells such as those in the gastrointestinal tract, bone marrow, and hair follicles. The killing of these cells leads to the side effects of gastrointestinal irritation, bone marrow depletion, and hair loss. The effects also vary in different patients. For some people, just knowing they will receive a dose of chemo causes anticipatory reactions such as vomiting.

The most common problems of chemotherapy, nausea and vomiting, often occur a few hours after it is administered and last only a short time. These problems can be greatly reduced by antinausea drugs that the chemotherapist can prescribe. These can be taken orally, intramuscularly, or rectally. Another common problem is the feeling of fatigue. Patients with this reaction must pace themselves and take rest periods during the day. Many patients do not feel tired at all and can continue their normal activities.

Despite the public's generally negative attitude toward chemotherapy, it is a powerful form of cancer treatment. Used either alone or in combination with surgery and radiation therapy, it has cured cancer in many patients and extended life, high-quality life, in many others.

Overview of Cancer Treatments

Surgical therapy cures more patients with cancer—of the breast, colon, prostate, uterus, cervix, and sometimes of the head and neck— than any other form of treatment. Surgery is not successful when the size of the cancer is too large or when the cancer has metastasized. Results of surgical therapy are improving because of new diagnostic techniques that more effectively pinpoint the extent of the cancer and because of the addition of radiation and chemotherapy to treat some patients.

Radiation therapy has an advantage over surgical therapy in that it may cause less cosmetic damage and impaired function, for instance, preservation of the voice in cancer of the larynx (voicebox). It, however, does not always reach the center of large tumors. Radiation therapy has been most successful in the treatment of Hodgkin's disease and prostate, cervical, and certain head and neck cancers. New advances in electronic and computer technology have allowed better localization of the margins of the tumors and more precise delivery of radiation to the tumor, minimizing exposure of adjacent normal tissues.

Chemotherapy has been most successful in the treatment of cancers with rapidly proliferating cells, such as acute leukemias, lymphomas, and testicular carcinomas. Chemotherapeutic drugs also kill rapidly dividing normal cells, though. The most prominent factor limiting their success in treating cancers is the capacity of selected cancer cells to become resistant to the action of the drugs. One current therapeutic strategy for certain leukemias and solid tumors attempts to sidestep both of these limitations to the use of chemotherapy: large doses of chemotherapeutic drugs along with total body irradiation, which together kill all the leukemic or cancer cells as well as the normal bone marrow cells. This is followed by transplantation to the patient of bone marrow obtained from the patient earlier, purged of cancer cells and stored until transplanted, or from appropriate donors.

In addition to surgery, radiation therapy, and chemotherapy used individually, their combined use has gradually evolved as a common treatment for certain cancers. Such combined therapy takes into account the usefulness as well as the limitation of each method. Surgery, while often curative in localized cancer, may fail to cure a patient because of undetected spread of the cancer cells beyond the margins of the surgical procedure. Radiation therapy is most effective for the treatment of the undetected disease at the margins of the excised tumor but is not, as just explained, effective in killing cancer cells in the center of large tumors. To circumvent these limitations, surgery can remove the large tumor, and radiation in lower doses can be used in a larger region surrounding the excised tumor. Chemotherapeutic drugs not useful for treatments of large tumors can then be used to kill residual cancer cells after these two therapies have removed the gross cancer and the local spread of cancer cells. Chemotherapy has also proved useful in reducing the size of large tumors, such as those in bladder cancers, so that they can be more easily removed by surgery. The three types of therapy have been successfully combined to treat breast cancer, sarcomas such as rhabdomyosarcomas of children, bone tumors, and a number of tumors of the head and neck.

While early diagnosis and modern treatment of these common cancers, with the exception of small-cell carcinoma of the lung, often lead to an extended high-quality life expectancy or cure, other cancers have a less optimistic prognosis. For instance, cancers of the pancreas, esophagus, and brain have a poor outlook, even with current therapy, as do advanced stages of the childhood cancer neuroblastoma.

Although the treatment programs described in this chapter for these major cancers are often successful and sometimes even curative, extensive efforts are under way to discover even more effective and less disfiguring or toxic treatments. Numerous clinical trials directed by the National Cancer Institute are being conducted, often on patients with recurrent cancer who volunteer to receive new, experimental forms of treatment. At the time of this writing, ninety-eight clinical trials are under way for recurrent breast cancer alone.

When Is Cancer Treatment Worthwhile?

This question has been posed since the advent of modern cancer treatment. In the early days, the question surrounded the hope for survival balanced against the pain and risks of major surgery. Now it has been expanded to include the hope for survival with an acceptable quality of life, against the risk and side effects of surgery, radiation therapy, chemotherapy, and other, more heroic treatments. It is still a difficult question to answer. In many types and stages of cancer, patients and their physicians must choose among treatments that will result in small differences in outcome. For instance, a patient may be asked to choose between a period of poor health due to surgery, radiation therapy, or chemotherapy followed by long, symptom-free survival and a shorter survival with no unpleasant side effects of treatment.

A young man with a testicular tumor may be willing to face surgery to remove the cancer followed by five weeks of radiation therapy and the associated nausea and vomiting in order to seek a cure. Studies have indicated that a large number of people with operable lung cancer choose radiation therapy alone to avoid the risks and discomfort associated with surgery, even though surgery may hold out the promise of a longer life (Tannock and Boyer 1990, p. 989). On the other hand, some women with breast cancer are willing to receive chemotherapy and accept the associated toxicity even though the gain in anticipated survival is small.

One major factor in the decision may be the cost. Economic analyses of combined therapy for some cancers indicate that it is cost-effective. For instance, the addition of chemotherapy for non-small-cell lung cancer, while it usually causes toxic side effects, does not always add expense because the cost of the drugs is offset by the shorter hospital stay.

Each patient, with help from family and close friends, as well as the most up-to-date information from enlightened physicians, must ultimately decide what type of cancer therapy, if any, he or she wants to receive. The options for treatments that lead to a cure or at least a prolonged survival with a high quality of life are immensely greater than ever before and will undoubtedly increase even further with the avalanche of new knowledge about the disease.

For More Information

A marvelous source of up-to-date information about cancer treatment is the Physician Data Query computer system (PDQ), a resource of the National Cancer Institute that is available not only to physicians and other health professionals but also to cancer patients and their families. PDQ describes the current treatments for most cancers and includes detailed descriptions of over 1,300 clinical trials entering new patients and more than 5,000 closed clinical trials. Also included is a directory of doctors who treat cancer and hospitals that have cancer programs. The information in PDQ is reviewed and updated by cancer experts every month. Because the current pace of research in cancer treatment is so fast, the information in the PDQ system is invaluable.

To contact PDQ for information about cancer, patients, families of patients, or physicians can call the National Cancer Institute's Cancer Information Service at its toll-free number: 1-800-422-6237. A trained counselor will talk to the caller, answer questions, and send free booklets. A new method for obtaining information in the PDQ computer system has been called "Getting the 'FAX' " on cancer treatments. By combining computer and facsimile (fax) technology, the National Cancer Institute created "Cancer FAX," a service that enables the NCI to send the information in PDQ to any physician with a fax machine. The service operates twenty-four hours a day, seven days a week, and is free of charge except for the cost of the telephone call to the Cancer fax computer in Bethesda, Maryland, at 301-402-5874. A recorded voice tells the caller how to obtain one of two printed statements about the treatment for seventy-nine cancers. One statement is more detailed and is intended for physicians. The other is written in language geared to be easily understood by the patient and is shorter, usually four pages in length.

Other important sources of information about cancer treatment and services are also available. The American Cancer Society, for instance, is an important resource for information about treatment care at home, transportation to and from places of treatment, and how to deal with the numerous problems associated with cancer.

Chapter 8

Clinical Trials

A CLINICAL TRIAL IS A STUDY THAT USES NEW TREATMENTS TO CARE for patients, usually an evaluation of a new cancer drug. Since the 1950s, thousands of potentially useful chemotherapeutic agents have been screened, or tested, in cultures of cancer cells, in experimental animals, and eventually in patients with cancer. It takes several years of step-by-step clinical trials for a new cancer drug that looks promising in the laboratory to be approved for general use. The average time between discovery and marketing of an antitumor agent is ten to twelve years.

Before a new drug can be used in clinical trials with cancer patients, the Food and Drug Administration must license it as an Investigational New Drug. The National Cancer Institute coordinates these clinical trials using investigators/doctors who participate on a voluntary basis. According to the National Cancer Institute, each year about 50,000 materials are tested, including chemical agents, antibiotics, natural products, and newly synthesized compounds. Only about 1 of every 5,000 agents screened in the laboratory is considered promising and safe enough to be tested on patients.

Following preclinical testing in cell cultures, rodents, and other animals, those drugs deemed possibly useful go through four phases of clinical testing in patients before they are accepted for general medical practice (see table 8.1).

Phase I trials are done on small groups of patients, usually no more than fifteen to thirty patients per study. Participating patients must

TABLE 8.1 *Stages in Clinical Testing of New Anticancer Agents*

Stages of Drug Testing	Objectives	Patient Population
Phase I	Determine largest tolerable dose of drug and dose schedule. Note reversibility of toxicity. Note therapeutic effect.	Advanced malignancy. Diagnosis clearly established. No longer amenable to conventional therapy. Stable health. Variety of cancer types permissible.
Phase II	Determine dose required to cause therapeutic effect in panel of cancers. Are toxic effects tolerable in relationship to therapeutic effect and in comparison to standard therapy?	Same as Phase I, plus measurable tumor masses, variety of tumor types in groups of 15–30 patients.
Phase III	Compare experimental therapy to standard therapy. Are toxic effects tolerable in relationship to therapeutic effect and in comparison to standard therapy?	Usually previously untreated. Diagnosis clearly established. Patient sample of adequate size and uniformity. Controls usually selected randomly but can be "historical" (previously treated patients).
Phase IV	Incorporation of new drug therapy into primary treatment in combination with surgery and/or radiation therapy. Compare to current standard therapy. Long-term toxic effects need monitoring (second cancers, sterility, bone marrow depletion).	Specific diagnosis. Large and uniform patient sample. Controls usually selected randomly.

give informed consent and make themselves available for close observation during the first few treatments. These patients have advanced cancers and have exhausted other forms of treatment but are in relatively good health. The main purpose of Phase I trials is to determine the highest dose that can be tolerated with the hope that some therapeutic effect will be achieved. Most drugs that go on to be marketed show some therapeutic effect even in Phase I trials. These trials are usually begun at one-tenth the dose that produced side effects in previous animal studies. The dose is then increased in succeeding groups of patients (usually three in a group) until toxicity is noted. Effects on the cancer are carefully observed. The data collected in this phase will indicate the side effects that can be expected in humans.

Phase II trials are designed to determine the responses of patients with specific cancers to a particular drug. These trials are again conducted in patients with advanced disease for whom no effective treatment is available, but who are otherwise relatively healthy. The anticancer activity of the drug is determined in groups of fifteen to thirty patients with several specific cancers. Tumor masses are measured and X-ray studies are made so that the effectiveness (shrinkage of the tumor) can be evaluated. The types of cancer that respond to the drug are closely evaluated to determine how useful various dosages are and how frequently they must be administered to obtain the best results.

At the completion of a Phase II trial, it must be decided whether to proceed to Phase III trials or to discard the drug. The decision is based on the observed therapeutic effect of the drug in relationship to excessive or intolerable toxicity.

Phase III trials use drugs found to be effective in Phase II trials. Now it must be determined whether the experimental drug is more useful and less toxic than other drugs currently used in standard therapy. The patients selected for these trials have usually had no previous treatment. These trials require large numbers of patients— 60 to 150 or more—with uniform types of cancer.

Phase IV trials integrate the experimental drug into initial treatment of a cancer patient in combination with surgery and/or radiation therapy. The purpose is to compare the new treatment program using the experimental drug with standard treatment programs. As in Phase III, large numbers of previously untreated patients with uniform types of cancer are required.

To make new drugs available to desperately ill cancer patients while this testing is under way, the NCI offers them to certain physicians as follows:

GROUP A DRUGS	These drugs are distributed by the NCI only to clinical investigators for use in Phase I and Phase II clinical trials in specific cancers.
GROUP B DRUGS	These drugs have been tested in Phase II clinical trials and are deemed to be possibly useful. The drugs are distributed more widely to Cancer Centers, Clinical Cooperative Groups, and NCI contractors.
GROUP C DRUGS	These drugs have demonstrated usefulness for at least one type of cancer and can be administered safely by properly trained physicians. These physicians must be registered with the NCI as investigators and must submit written requests for the drug, stating which cancer is to be treated.

The use of the drugs is limited to indications for use listed in guidelines that are provided to the physician. The physician must report all adverse reactions caused by the drug to the Investigational Drug Branch of the NCI.

A patient may receive an experimental anticancer drug only after the potential value and potential risks have been carefully explained and he or she has signed a consent form. The patient and the family should weigh the possible advantages of the treatment against the problems it might cause. The patient must qualify under very specific criteria, including a precise diagnosis obtained by microscopic examination of a biopsy of the tumor, as well as X ray and possibly other studies to determine the extent of the disease and the overall health of the patient. The experimental anticancer drugs are available only to physicians using them under the auspices of the National Cancer Institute and following specific U.S. Food and Drug Administration regulations for their use. As described earlier, before being tested on cancer patients, all drugs have passed rigorous preclinical testing and evaluation.

Only qualified oncologists (cancer specialists) are allowed to administer investigational cancer drugs. Further, the use of the drugs must follow specific written guidelines, or protocols, which describe the overall treatment plan for their use. Such protocols include the criteria for selecting patients, the dose time and route of administration of the drug (oral or intravenous, for example), as well as requirements for collecting and reporting information on the patients.

For Phases III and IV, the patients must be informed that they have been selected randomly (randomized) on an unbiased basis into groups, or "arms," some of whom will be given the new drug and others, the standard therapy. Neither the patient nor the doctor knows which group the patient has been "randomized" to, in an effort to remove bias on the part of the doctors and to establish clearly whether one treatment is better than the other. Such studies are called "double-blind." In some of the studies, however, both the patient and the physician know which drugs are being used.

All patients participating in NCI-sponsored clinical trials are protected by regulations of the Department of Health and Human Services pertaining to studies with human subjects. The Cancer Center or other institution in which the trials are conducted must have an Institutional Review Board (IRB) consisting of medical scientists and local community members (who have no formal relationship to the institution), who receive all available information about the proposed treatment plan and judge whether the importance of the new information about cancer treatment to be obtained outweighs the risks to the patient.

In addition, the IRB members review the proposed informed-consent forms that will be submitted to the patient to be certain they are written in language understandable to a lay person. Before a patient (or family member, for young children) agrees to an experimental treatment and signs the informed consent, his or her physician will have gone over the following:

- A thorough explanation of the treatment to be followed
- A description of the possible toxic reaction and risks to be expected
- A disclosure of alternate treatment plans that might be advantageous to the patient
- A notification that the patient is free to withdraw consent and to discontinue participation in the treatment program at any time.

The costs of anticancer drugs vary according to the drugs being used, how often they are administered, and what institution is carrying out the clinical trial. Physicians' fees and laboratory tests may also add to the costs of the therapy. Some medical insurance policies cover some of these costs, but the patient or family should find out ahead of time so they know exactly what the trial will cost them.

Patients who wish to learn about clinical trials for their type of cancer can call the National Cancer Institute's Cancer Information Service 1-800-4-CANCER. A trained counselor will answer their questions about their cancer and clinical trials for its treatment. Also available are lists of many doctors who take part in clinical trials and a free booklet, *What Are Clinical Trials All About?* Patients or their families can also write to the National Cancer Institute at Building 31, Room 10A24, 9000 Rockville Pike, Bethesda, Maryland 20892.

The remainder of this chapter is devoted to a reprinting of a report of a specific clinical trial, submitted by the Principal Investigator, Steven A. Rosenberg, M.D., PH.D., to the Clinical Research Subpanel of the NCI (equivalent to an IRB). It lists the objectives, rationale or basis for the trial, type of patient eligible, plan for treatment, evaluation of various effects of treatment, and possible side effects or adverse reactions. Also noted is that if no responses are detected in the first fourteen patients treated, "no further patients with that histologic type of cancer will be admitted to the protocol."

The "Consent to Participate in a Clinical Research Study" points out that taking part in the study is entirely voluntary and that patients may withdraw from it at any time. The informed-consent form describes the study, its risks, its inconveniences, and other information. It encourages the patient to discuss the study and to ask questions of the staff, whose names, addresses, and phone numbers are provided. Cancer patients are not paid for taking part in NIH studies, but there may be exceptions to this rule, as guided by clinical center policies. All participants must sign an approved informed consent in the presence of one of the investigators and a witness.

Initial Proposal of Clinical Research Project

Date: March 25, 1991   Clinical Project Number: 91-C-163
To: Chairman, Clinical Research Subpanel, NCI
Recommended by:

_____, Deputy Clinical
Director, NCI

_____, Branch Chief(s)

Immunization of Cancer Patients Using Autologous Cancer Cells Modified by Insertion of the Gene for Tumor Necrosis Factor

Identifying Words: gene therapy, immunotherapy, interleukin-2, tumor infiltrating lymphocytes, tumor necrosis factor

PRINCIPAL
INVESTIGATOR: Steven A. Rosenberg, M.D., Ph.D.
ASSOCIATE
INVESTIGATORS: W. F. Anderson, M.D., Molecular Hematology
                    Branch, NHLBI
                  A. L. Asher, M.D., Surgery Branch, NCI
                  M. R. Blaese, Cellular Immunology Section, MB,
                    NCI
                  S. E. Ettinghausen, M.D., Surgery Branch, NCI
                  P. Hwu, M.D., Surgery Branch, NCI
                  A. Kasid, Ph.D., Surgery Branch, NCI
                  J. J. Mule, Ph.D., Surgery Branch, NCI
                  D. R. Parkinson, M.D., Cancer Therapy Evaluation
                    Program
                  D. J. Schwartzentruber, M.D., Surgery Branch, NCI
                  S. L. Topalian, M.D., Surgery Branch, NCI
                  J. S. Weber, M.D., Surgery Branch, NCI
                  J. R. Yannelli, Ph.D., Surgery Branch, NCI
                  J. C. Yang, M.D., Surgery Branch, NCI
                  W. M. Linehan, M.D., Surgery Branch, NCI

Estimated Duration of Study: 3 years

Number and Kind of Subjects Needed:	Number	Sex (M or F)	Age
Patients	50	M&F	18 & older

Precis: When tumor is resected from patients as part of the natural course of their treatment, an attempt will be made to establish a tissue culture line of the tumor.

The gene coding for tumor necrosis factor will be introduced into these tumor cells and the integration and expression of this gene will be tested. Patients will become eligible for this study only if they develop metastatic cancer that has failed all standard effective treatment and have no other effective treatment options available to them. Tumor cells will be injected intradermally and subcutaneously into the thigh of these patients. The amount of tumor injected will be less than $1/50$th the total tumor burden of the patient. In previous studies we have shown that these gene-modified tumor cells are more immunogenic than the native unaltered tumor. Attempts will then be made to grow immune lymphocytes either from the tumor site or from the draining lymph nodes of these patients in order to use these lymphocytes for adoptive immunotherapy as detailed in previous protocols. The direct effect of the immunization with these immunogenic tumor cells will also be measured by assessing the impact on established tumor at other sites. Fifty patients receiving tumor inoculation will be included in this study.

I. Objectives

To evaluate the possible therapeutic efficacy of the injection of autologous cancer cells modified by insertion of the gene for tumor necrosis factor into patients with advanced cancer.

II. Introduction and Rationale

1. *Cell Transfer Therapy Using TIL.* Research in the Surgery Branch, NCI, has been directed toward developing new immunotherapies for the treatment of patients with cancer (1–5). Based on extensive animal experimentation we developed treatment approaches using the administration of high-dose interleukin-2 (IL-2) alone or in conjunction with the adoptive transfer of lymphokine activated killer (LAK) cells in patients with advanced cancer (1). We have now treated 178 patients using LAK cells in conjunction with IL-2 and 136 patients with high dose IL-2 alone (3). These studies have demonstrated that the administration of high-dose IL-2, either alone or in conjunction with LAK cells, can result in the regression of advanced cancer in some patients. Approximately 10% of patients with metastatic renal cell cancer and melanoma will undergo a complete regression of cancer following treatment with LAK cells and IL-2 and an additional 10–25% of patients will undergo an objective partial remission.

In an attempt to improve upon these results, we identified and characterized a more potent type of killer cell called the tumor infiltrating lymphocyte (TIL) (6). These cells are cytolytic T lymphocytes. In both mice and human TIL can develop the ability to specifically lyse the syngeneic or autologous tumor and not normal cells or allogeneic tumors (7,8). We demonstrated that TIL were from 50–100 times more potent on a per cell basis than were LAK cells in mediating the regression of established cancer in several murine tumor models (6). These animal experiments led to clinical trials of the use of TIL in humans (5). Thirty-eight percent of melanoma patients underwent an objective regression of their cancer; however, the duration of responses has been variable and in many cases this response has been of short duration.

Extensive studies have been performed in the Surgery Branch, NCI, to study the characteristics of human TIL and the mechanism of action of these cells in patients (9). In an attempt to study the traffic of TIL following cell infusion, 19 infusions of TIL labeled with Indium-111 were given to 18 patients and the distribution of these cells assessed using gamma camera imaging and sequential biopsies (10). Clear tumor localization of TIL was seen on 13 of 18 nuclear scan series and sequential biopsy data confirmed the homing of TIL to tumor deposits. These findings raised the possibility that TIL might be used as vehicles to deliver, to the tumor site, molecules that might enhance the antitumor activity of the TIL transfer.

To further study the distribution and survival of TIL we have performed studies of the retroviral transduction of the gene coding for neomycin resistance into TIL (11) and the subsequent infusion of these TIL into 10 autologous patients with advanced cancer (2). Extensive studies have been conducted on the first five patients. No toxicities of any kind could be attributed to the gene modification of the TIL. The expected toxicities associated with the concomitant administration of IL-2 were seen. Patients received up to 1.45×10^{11} gene-transduced TIL populations. The percent of cells transduced in these populations varied between 1 and 11%. In all cases, integration and expression of the NeoR gene was demonstrated. Gene modified TIL could be detected at tumor deposits as long as 64 days after gene transduction.

All safety studies performed in these patients showed no evidence of exposure to replication competent virus. 3T3 amplification and S +/L − assays revealed no replication competent virus present in the TIL at the time they were infused. Polymerase chain reaction analysis for the viral envelope gene and reverse transcriptase assay of the gene-modified TIL culture were also negative. Western blot analyses of patient serum at various times after cell administration were all negative for evidence of exposure to virus as well. These studies demonstrated that gene modification of the TIL could be performed and that these TIL could be infused with no exposure of the patient to a replication competent virus. These studies provided us with valuable experience to perform subsequent studies of TIL modified with the gene for tumor necrosis factor (TNF). These studies began on January 29, 1991, and thus far two patients have been treated with escalating doses of TIL transduced with the gene for TNF. Thus far no side effects have been seen in these two patients.

2. *Tumor Necrosis Factor.* The injection of recombinant TNF can mediate the necrosis and regression of a variety of established experimental murine cancers (13–15). The combined administration of TNF and IL-2 mediated far greater antitumor effects against subcutaneous and liver tumors than either cytokine alone (16). The exact mechanisms of TNF antitumor effects are not clearly understood, although it appears that TNF has a significant effect on the vascular supply of tumors and CD8 + cells (15). Membrane-bound TNF may be involved in direct tumor lysis as well (17). These animal experiments have led to extensive tests of recombinant human TNF administered to humans with advanced cancer (3,18–21). In the Surgery Branch, NCI, we treated 38 patients with advanced cancer using escalating doses of recombinant TNF (supplied by the Cetus Corp., Emeryville, California) administered in conjunction with IL-2 (3). No antitumor effects of TNF administration have been seen in humans. However, when high local

concentrations of TNF are achieved at tumor sites by direct intralesional TNF rejection, tumor regression in humans has been seen.

Extensive studies of the difference between the dramatic response of mice to the systemic injection of TNF and the lack of effect in humans have focused on the substantial differences in tolerance of mice and man to the administration of TNF. Tumor-bearing mice can tolerate from 400–500 µg/kg TNF and these doses are required to mediate tumor regression; the administration of less TNF is far less effective (15). In contrast, the maximum tolerated dose of TNF in both Surgery Branch, NCI, and other studies is approximately 8 µg/kg/day. Thus when injected intravenously only 2% of the TNF dose required to mediate antitumor effects in the mouse can be administered to man.

Because of the unique effectiveness of TNF in the treatment of a variety of murine malignancies, we have sought means to selectively increase the local concentration of TNF at the tumor site. Because TIL can traffic directly to tumor deposits and concentrate at those sites, we hypothesized that TIL transduced with the gene for TNF and producing large amounts of TNF in the local tumor microenvironment might have substantially increased antitumor effects compared to normal TIL. This hypothesis served as the basis for the protocol dealing with the administration of TIL transduced with the gene for TNF that is now underway.

In the course of these studies we used retroviral vectors to introduce the gene coding for TNF into murine and human tumors. These transduced tumor cell lines produced up to 15 ng TNF/10^6 cells/24 hours. Extensive studies introducing the TNF gene construct into human melanoma cell lines were similar. These transduced cells contained one to two copies per cell of an unrearranged TNF vector genome and expressed transcripts homologous to the TNF cDNA corresponding to the proviral transcribed full-length message. The human tumor cell lines produced up to 15 ng TNF/10^6 cells/24 hr.

Extensive experiments were performed to test the immunogenicity of these tumor lines in both syngeneic mice as well as in nude mice. In murine models we found that unmodified parenteral tumor cells grew aggressively when implanted subcutaneously into syngeneic mice, although tumor cells transduced with the TNF gene regressed in a significant number of animals after an initial phase of growth. This effect correlated with the amount of TNF produced and could be blocked with a specific anti-TNF antibody. The regression of these TNF-producing cells was not associated with any demonstrable toxicity in the mice bearing these tumors.

The increased immunogenicity of these TNF-producing tumor cells was demonstrated by experiments showing the immunologic nature of this tumor regression. TNF-producing tumor cells grew well in irradiated mice but not in non-irradiated mice. Further, the ability of tumor cells to regress was abrogated by depletion of the CD8+ T cell subset. Further, animals that experienced regression of TNF-producing tumors rejected a subsequent challenge of unmodified tumor indicating the state of immunity to the tumor that had regressed. In addition, TNF-producing tumor cells could function in a paracrine fashion by inhibiting the growth of unmodified tumor cells implanted at the same site. It thus appears from these murine studies that tumor cells elaborating high local concentrations of TNF could regress in the absence of toxicity in the host and that this regression was immunologically mediated.

Similar studies were performed using TNF gene–modified human tumor cells injected into athymic nude mice. Following the injection of 4 to 8 × 10⁶ human tumor cells into nude mice, non-transduced or neomycin-transduced tumor cells grew progressively. However, tumors that were transduced with the TNF gene stopped growing after 8 to 10 days in all of the animals and complete tumor regression was seen in some of the mice. In these experiments, DNA was extracted from some stable or regressing human tumors, and Southern analysis revealed intact, unrearranged proviral DNA present in all the regressing tumors induced by TNF-transduced cells. The proviral sequences were undetectable in the proliferating tumors formed by the non-transduced cells. The paracrine function of the TNF produced by human tumors was also seen. The localized elaboration of TNF by TNF-transduced cells was also effective in suppressing tumor formation by control NeoR-transduced cells injected at the same site.

It thus appears that in syngeneic mice the injection of TNF-modified tumor cells was more immunogenic than unmodified cells and could induce an immunity sufficient to cause the regression of these TNF gene–modified tumor cells as well as normal tumor cells mixed at the same site. In this proposal we thus plan to take advantage of the increased immunogenicity of these TNF-producing tumors to attempt to immunize patients with advanced and otherwise untreatable metastatic cancer. These tumor cells will be injected subcutaneously and intradermally into the thigh in an area that can be followed easily in an attempt to both immunize the patient against their cancer as well as to provide local immunization that could be used to grow lymphocytes for use in adoptive therapy. Lymphocytes will be obtained either from the draining inguinal lymph node group or from the tumor site itself.

In addition to the increased immunogenicity of the gene-modified tumor, recent work in the Surgery Branch has suggested that the subcutaneous injection of tumor can lead to the development of more effective tumor-infiltrating lymphocytes. In 12 successive experiments, TIL grown from visceral sites were simultaneously tested by careful *in vivo* titration against TIL from tumor injected into the cutaneous site. In 11 of 12 experiments, TIL from the subcutaneous location were more effective than those at visceral sites. In three other experiments, TIL from murine tumors in the liver were less effective than TIL from cutaneous sites.

In the human, other workers have shown that small cutaneous tumor auto inoculations can provoke significant immune responses. Hoover and Hanna have published work in which colorectal cancers from primary sites were irradiated and utilized for autologous immunization of patients in the adjuvant setting (22). Patients with Dukes B2 and C tumors demonstrated improved overall survival in a randomized study, presumably due to an effective immune response to the immunization. In addition, Berg and Mastrangelo have investigated the immunization of melanoma patients with irradiated autologous tumor, and have demonstrated the induction of significant T-cell infiltrates in tumors as well as rare clinical responses in patients with metastatic disease (23,24). These studies generally utilized irradiated tumor cell inoculation and therefore result in no tumor for the generation of TIL. The presence of tumor is vital for generating optimal TIL in that T-cells separated from fresh tumors will grow in vitro with IL-2 but will show decreased in vivo efficacy if not re-exposed to tumor in culture (presumably due to the requirement of cultured T-cells for antigen exposure) (25). Furthermore, irradiated or non-viable tumor and tumor extracts produce immune responses in animals that are typically inferior to the responses to viable tumor (26). Therefore the injection of small amounts of viable tumor at a cutaneous site might not only result in tumor for TIL production, but also generate an immune response superior to that demonstrated using irradiated or non-viable tumor. This immune response may not only be seen at the tumor site, but pre-clinical models show that T-cells can be recovered in lymph nodes draining the site of tumor inoculation, which can be expanded in culture and show in vivo antitumor activity. This aspect of the cellular immune response to tumor immunization will be discussed later in the protocol.

Because tumor growth at the transplant site is necessary for TIL production, it is important to know if that will occur and what are the potential risks involved. Southam and Brunschwig inoculated a series of patients with a variety of metastatic cancers with their own resected tumors in graded doses (27,28). This revealed that the majority of patients could grow tumors at these inoculation sites if an adequate inoculum was administered. These were all patients with widely metastatic disease or unresectable advanced cancers, and no impact from the inoculations on their overall clinical course was identified. For patients with widely metastatic cancer, a very small local cutaneous tumor inoculation (representing a fraction of their progressive metastatic disease) and subsequent resection of any growing tumor is unlikely to significantly accelerate the course of their systemic disease. In support of this, one can cite the extreme case of tumor auto-inoculation which occurs when large numbers of malignant cells are intravenously infused as a result of peritoneal-venous shunting to palliate malignant ascites. Multiple clinical and post-mortem studies fail to show significant decreases in survival or alterations in the pattern of metastatic disease in shunted versus non-shunted patients (29–31). Such shunted patients can develop microscopic metastatic implantation, but these studies show that these implants fail to reach a significant size prior to the patient's death from their pre-existing known metastatic disease. Certainly the cells which might escape from a small, cutaneously implanted tumor site into the systemic circulation (if this occurs at all) would be far less than that from the intravenous auto-innoculation which occurs on a daily basis in these shunted patients or in any patient with widely metastatic cancer.

Thus, data suggests that auto-inoculation of a small amount of viable tumor at an isolated cutaneous site will often generate tumors for TIL growth, but that in the setting of widely metastatic cancer, such an approach is unlikely to significantly affect survival or the disease course of such patients. In the experiments in this protocol, however, the introduction of the TNF gene into tumor is designed to increase the immunogenicity of the tumor (as reviewed earlier) and will prevent tumor growth in most cases. The use of draining lymph node lymphocytes can thus provide a source of cells for use in adoptive immunotherapy of these patients.

Shu et al. have published data in murine models showing that draining lymph node lymphocytes (DLNL) from sites of tumor immunization can be sensitized in vitro (by mixed tumor-lymphocyte culture) and expanded in IL-2 (32–34). These cells can then be adoptively transferred to tumor-bearing mice and show antitumor activity. Many of the features of these cells are similar to TIL (such as phenotype and tumor specificity patterns), although they have a lesser capability to expand in vitro and may be somewhat less effective on a cell-for-cell basis (25,35). These cultured draining lymph node cells are currently undergoing Phase I testing by Dr. Alfred Chang at the University of Michigan. In order to provide patients undergoing tumor immunization with a treatment alternative in the event of failure of the primary TIL culture, at the time of resection of inoculation sites (or at three weeks after inoculation if no tumor growth is apparent), draining lymph nodes will be excisionally biopsied to prepare an alternative T-cell culture for adoptive transfer. This will be performed with sensitization using autologous cryopreserved tumor (from the original source used for inoculation) and IL-2. These lymph node lymphocytes will be given with systemic IL-2 exactly as intended for TIL.

III. Patient Eligibility

The eligibility of patients for whom cell lines will be established and who will be offered the treatment portions of this protocol are the same and are listed below:

1. Patients, age 18 or older, must have histologically confirmed metastatic cancer for which standard curative or palliative measures do not exist or are no longer effective. These patients have expected survivals of six months or less.

2. The estimated tumor burden of the patient must be at least 10 grams, which is 50 times the weight of tumor cells used for the immunization.

3. Women of childbearing potential must have a negative pregnancy test.

4. Patients must have a negative HIV test.

5. Patients must have a performance status less than 2 and must be free of active systemic infections and other major medical illnesses of the cardiovascular and respiratory systems. They should have the following laboratory values:

    a. white blood cell count greater than $3000/mm^3$
    b. platelet count greater than $150,000/mm^3$
    c. bilirubin less than 1.7 mg/dl
    d. creatinine less than 1.7 mg/dl

6. Patients requiring steroid therapy will be excluded.

7. Patients who have received therapy with cytotoxic agents, steroids, other biologics, or radiotherapy in the 4 weeks prior to cell inoculation will be excluded.

IV. Treatment Plan

1. *Summary.* Tissue culture lines will be established from resected tumors during the course of normal patient treatment. The gene for tumor necrosis factor will be inserted into these tumor cells using either retroviral mediated gene transduction or by transfection techniques using calcium phosphate or microinjection. Patients that develop advanced untreatable metastatic cancer and have failed all other effective treatments will be offered the possibility of joining this protocol. After signing an informed consent the patients will be registered in the protocol and will receive the injection of the gene-modified tumor cells into the mid thigh. Up to 2×10^8 gene-modified tumor cells will be injected in 1 ml subcutaneously and three centimeters lateral or vertical from this site the patient will receive two intradermal injections of 2×10^7 gene-modified tumor cells in 0.1 ml each. These sites will then be carefully monitored. At three weeks the patient will undergo resection of several lymph nodes from the draining superficial inguinal area. These

lymph nodes will be used to grow lymphocytes for adoptive cellular therapy of that patient. As predicted by animal models, it is not expected that tumor will grow at the local injection site. If, however, tumor does grow, then the soft tissue in the area of the tumor injection will be resected when a tumor has reached one to two centimeters and an attempt will be made to grow tumor-infiltrating lymphocytes from this site. Lymphocytes either from draining lymph nodes or from the tumor site itself (whichever become available first) will be grown in vitro by the standard techniques used in many previous protocols and assays published in detail. These lymphocytes will then be adoptively transferred to the patient along with 720,000 IU/kg of IL-2, exactly as in our previous protocols and as previously published in detail. The impact of the immunization procedure on established tumor at other sites will also be monitored to evaluate whether this immunization procedure itself has antitumor effects. Biopsies of cutaneous or subcutaneous lesions may be performed.

2. *Preparation of the TNF-NeoR Vector Containing Supernatant.* The TNF-NeoR vector used in this protocol is identical to that used in our approved protocol (#90-C-186) utilizing the introduction of these genes into human tumor-infiltrating lymphocytes for use in human therapy. The following description of the vector containing supernatant is taken verbatim from that approved protocol.

The TNF-NeoR vector was constructed by modifying the Moloney murine leukemia vector by techniques similar to those previously described. Retroviral vector supernatant is produced by harvesting the cell culture medium from the PA317 packaging line developed by Dr. A. Dusty Miller (36,37). This line has been extensively characterized and was used by us in our previous studies of the infusion of TIL modified by the LNL6 vector (11,12). The TNF-Neo vector preparations from PA317 will be extensively tested to assure that no detectable replication competent virus is present. Tests for replication competent virus will be conducted on both the vector supernatant and on the tumor cells after transduction. The vector includes the retroviral LTR promoting the TNF gene followed by the SV-40 early promoter and the gene coding for neomycin phosphotransferase. Testing will be the same as previously approved for the LNL6 supernatants used to introduce the NeoR gene into TIL (protocol 86-C-183c). The following tests will be run on the producer line and/or the viral supernatant:

1) The viral titer will be determined on 3T3 cells. Viral preparations with titers greater than 5×10^4 colony forming units/ml will be used.

2) Southern blots will be run on the producer line to detect the TNF gene.

3) TNF production by the producer line will be measured and should be significantly above baseline control values. TNF will be assayed using standard biologic assays on the L929 sensitive cell line (15) or by ELISA assay (R&D Systems, Minneapolis, MN).

4) Sterility of the producer line and the supernatant will be assured by testing for aerobic and anaerobic bacteria, fungus, and for mycoplasma.

5) Viral testing will be performed including:
   a. MAP test
   b. LCM virus
   c. Thymic agent
   d. S+/L− assay for ecotropic virus
   e. S+/L− for xenotropic virus

    f. S+/L− for amphotropic virus

    g. 3T3 amplification

  6) Electron microscopy will be performed to assure the absence of adventitious agents.

The retroviral supernatant will not be used to transduce tumor cells injected into patients until approval is received from the Food and Drug Administration.

    3. *Preparation of Gene-Modified Tumor Cells.* Tumor lines will be established in tissue culture from tumor fragments or single cell suspensions using standard tissue culture techniques (38). Tumor and normal tissue will be obtained immediately after surgery and processed as follows. The tumors were minced into 1 mm³ fragments and dissociated with agitation in serum-free DMEM (Dulbecco Modified Eagle Medium) (Biofluids) containing 2 mM glutamine, 0.1 mg/ml hyaluronidase, 0.02 mg/ml Dnase I and 0.1 mg/ml collagenase for 3 hours at room temperature. The cell suspension was then centrifuged at 800 g for 5 minutes and the pellet resuspended in a culture medium consisting of 5 ml of DMEM high glucose (4.5 g/l) with penicillin and glutamine supplemented with 10% fetal calf serum. The cells were either centrifuged prior to being frozen in 90% FCS, 10% DMSO at −80°C, or plated in appropriate dishes or culture flasks in culture medium. Plated cells were incubated at 37°C in a humidified atmosphere of 5% CO₂ and 95% air. Within 48 hrs, the culture medium was changed in order to remove all non-attached material. Subsequently, cultures were incubated for a period of 6 to 8 days without medium change. The tumors grow as adherent monolayers in tissue culture flasks (Falcon #3028; 175 cm²; 750 ml) containing about 50 ml of medium. When the cells are actively growing and not yet confluent, the medium will be poured off and 30–50 ml of medium containing the retroviral supernatant with 5 µg/ml protamine will be added to the flask (39). The flasks will be incubated at 37°C for six hours, at which time the medium will be changed. This procedure will be repeated up to three times. After 24 to 48 hours medium containing 300 µg/ml G418 will be added directly to the flask and the cells will be grown and subcultured for 7 to 14 days in G418 containing medium. The G418 concentration may be raised to 1 mg/ml depending on the health of the culture.

    4. *Tests on the Transduced Tumor Population.* Following transduction, growth, and selection of the tumor populations, the following tests will be performed on the tumor prior to injection into patients.

  1) Cell viability will be greater than 70% as tested by trypan dye exclusion.

  2) Sterility will be assured by testing for aerobic and anaerobic bacteria, fungus, and mycoplasma.

  3) S+/L− assay must be negative.

  4) Southern blot or PCR analysis will be run on the transduced tumor to assure that proviral sequences are present.

  5) TNF protein assay to assure the production of TNF. Cells must be producing at least 100 pg TNF/10⁶ cells/24 hours.

The S+/L− assay, the 3T3 amplification assay and the polymerase chain reaction assay are detailed in the Appendix.

    5. *Injection of Tumor Cells.* Gene-modified tumor cells will be harvested from the culture flasks by exposure to 0.25% versene (EDTA) for 10 minutes. The cells will be washed three times by suspension in 50 mls normal saline and centrifu-

gation. The final cell pellet will be suspended in normal saline and counted. 2×10^8 viable cells in 1 ml normal saline will be injected subcutaneously just beneath the skin in the anterior mid thigh and the overlying skin marked with a tattoo dot. If 2×10^8 cells are not available, fewer may be given but not less than 2×10^7 cells will be injected. About 3 cm lateral or vertical to this injection the patient will receive two intradermal injections (separated by 1 cm) of 2×10^7 gene-modified tumor cells in 0.1 ml normal saline and these sites also marked by a tattoo dot. These sites will be monitored weekly by a physician. At three weeks the patient will undergo excisional biopsy of superficial inguinal lymph nodes (without formal dissection) in the area draining the inoculation site for growth of lymphocytes. If tumor grows at any of these sites they will be excised when they reach 1 to 2 cm for growth of TIL. If no tumor growth is evident then the sites of tumor injection will be excisionally biopsied at 8 weeks after injection for pathologic analysis.

6. *Growth of Lymphocytes.* The procedures used here are the same as those used in our previous protocols (40) involving the infusion of TIL (86-C-183) and are taken virtually verbatim from that protocol.

At least two days prior to surgery, peripheral blood lymphocytes are collected by leukapheresis for four hours. These are Ficoll-Hypaque separated and the mononuclear cells collected from the interface, washed in saline, and placed in culture in roller bottles at 10^6 cells/ml. Half are placed into AIMV (a serum-free medium, Gibco Laboratories) with 6000 IU/ml IL-2 (Cetus), and half are placed into RPMI supplemented with 2% type-compatible human serum, penicillin (unless the patient is allergic), gentamicin, and 6000 IU/ml IL-2. After 3 to 4 days cells are centrifuged and the supernatants are collected and filtered. These are referred to as LAK supernatants.

Immediately upon resection of tumor or lymph nodes, the specimen(s) is transported to the laboratory in a sterile container and placed on a sterile dissection board in a laminar flow hood. A small representative portion is taken for pathologic analysis, and the rest is minced into pieces roughly 4 mm in diameter. These are placed into an enzyme solution of collagenase, DNAse type I, and hyaluronidase type V as previously described for overnight digestion at room temperature. The resulting suspension is filtered through a wire mesh to remove any large debris, washed in saline, and placed on Ficoll-Hypaque gradients. The interface containing viable lymphocytes is collected and washed in saline, and a portion is frozen for subsequent use as targets in cytotoxicity assays.

Lymphocyte cultures are initiated at 5×10^5 ml viable cells in 80% fresh medium/20% LAK supernatant. For half the cells, the fresh medium is AIMV supplemented with penicillin, fungizone, and 6000 IU/ml IL-2; for the other half, the fresh medium is RPMI supplemented with 10% human serum, penicillin, streptomycin, gentamicin, fungizone, and 6000 IU/ml IL-2. The cultures are placed into 6-well tissue culture dishes and incubated at 37° in humidified incubators with 5% CO_2. Cultures initiated from lymph nodes will be cocultivated with cryopreserved tumor stimulation cells at an initial ratio of at least 1:10 tumor cells to lymphocytes (but not more than 1:1) depending on the availability of tumor cells.

Usually the lymphocyte density is not much increased at the end of seven days in culture, and the cultures are collected, centrifuged, and resuspended at 5×10^5 total viable cells/ml is newly prepared 80%/20% medium mixtures of the same type. Occasionally a culture will have increased lymphocyte density and need medium replenishment prior to seven days. After this first passage, lymphocytes are subcultured by dilution when the density is between 1.5×10^6 and 2.5×10^6 cells per ml; densities of subcultures are established between 3×10^5 and 6×10^5 ml. Cultures are kept in 6-well dishes when the volume is less than 1 liter, and transferred to 3 liter polyolefin bags (Fenwal) when the volume reaches one liter. The subcultures from bags are accomplished with Fluid Fill/Weigh Units (Fenwal), which are programmed to pump prescribed weights of TIL culture and fresh medium into a new bag. When subculture volumes exceed 3 liters, the fresh medium used in AIMV. Cultures growing in serum-containing medium are thus diluted into AIMV, and no further LAK supernatant is added to cultures growing in serum-containing or serum-free medium.

If, during the growth of TIL, patients performance status has deteriorated to 3 or greater or if they have developed significant cardiac, renal, pulmonary, or hematologic dysfunction, then they will be taken off study and will not receive the infusion of TIL or IL-2.

When the total lymphocytes for a patient are ready for harvest, 5×10^6 cells are taken from cytological examination. Cytospins are examined for the presence of remaining tumor. At least 200 cells are studied and therapy proceeds only when no tumor cells are found. Other lymphocyte samples are taken for characterization of cell surface markers and for assessment of cytotoxicity using techniques identical to that in our previous protocol (86-C-183; reference 23, attached). Briefly, lymphocytes are stained with fluorescent-labeled antibodies (Leu2, Leu3, Leu4, Leu7, Leu11, Leu5, Leu9, LeuM3, HLADDR, and Tac). Chromium release assays are performed with K562, Daudi autologous tumor, and allogeneic tumor targets.

To infuse the lymphocytes they will be thawed and grown for one to three additional weeks using the same procedures detailed above. For infusion TIL are reharvested. At the time of cell collection, one liter of saline for injection is pumped through the collection chamber and the centrifuge is stopped. Lymphocytes are resuspended in the collection bag, the centrifuge is started again, and another liter of saline is pumped through to fully wash the free of tissue culture medium components. The cells are then filtered through a platelet administration set into 600 ml transfer packs (Fenwal), and 50 ml of 25% albumin and 450,000 IU of IL-2 are added to the 200 to 300 ml volume of cells in saline. The TIL are infused over 30 to 60 minutes through a central venous catheter.

7. *Interleukin-2.* The recombinant IL-2 used in this trial will be provided by the Division of Cancer Treatment, National Cancer Institute (supplied by the Cetus Corporation, Emeryville, CA) (28) and will be administered exactly as specified in our previously approved protocols (86-C-183c) (41). The IL-2 will be provided as a lyophilized powder and will be reconstituted with 1.2 ml/vial. Each vial contains approximately 1.2 mg of IL-2 (specific activity 18×10^6 IV/mg). Less than 0.04 ng of endotoxin are present per vial as measured by the limulus amebocyte assay. Each vial also contains 5% mannitol and approximately 130–230 µg of sodium dodecyl sulfate/mg of IL-2. Following reconstitution the IL-2 will be diluted in 50 ml of normal saline containing 5% human serum albumin and will be infused intravenously at a dose of 720,000 IU/kg over a 15-minute period every 8 hr, beginning from two to 24 hr after the TIL infusion. IL-2 will be given for up to five consecutive days as tolerated. Under no circumstances will more than 15 doses of IL-2 be administered. The same toxicity criteria will be used as in our previous protocol

(86-C-183c). Doses may be skipped depending on patient tolerance. Doses will be skipped if patients reach grade III or grade IV toxicity. If this toxicity is easily reversed by supportive measures then additional doses may be given.

8. *Concomitant Therapy.* Patients may receive concomitant medications to control the side effects of therapy (4,5). It is our plan to administer the same concomitant medications used in all previous TIL protocols. These include: acetaminophen (650 mg every 4 hours), indomethacin (50–75 mg every six hours), and ranitidine (150 mg every 12 hours) throughout the course of treatment. Patients may receive intravenous meperidine (25–50 mg) to control chills when they occur, although chills are unusual after the first one to two doses of IL-2. Hydroxyzine hydrochloride (25 mg every six hours) is given to treat pruritis. Steroids will not be used in these patients and if steroids are required, then the patient will immediately be taken off protocol therapy.

V. Patient Evaluation

Parameters to Be Measured

	Pre Study	D1	D3	D5	During Therapy D6	D15	D17	D19	D20	Week 7
Physical exam	X				X					
History	X	X								X
Performance Status	X									X
Assess for Tumor Effect[1]	X	X	X	X	X	X	X	X	X	X
Chemistry Survey[2]	X	X	X	X	X	X	X	X	X	X
Vital Signs	X	X	X	X	X	X	X	X	X	
Weight	X	X	X	X	X	X	X	X	X	X
CBC, Diff, Platelet	X	X	X	X	X	X	X	X	X	X
PT, PTT	X	X		X		X		X		X
FEV1, ABGs	X									
EKG	X							X		X
CXR	X				X	X		X		X
Cardiac Stress Test	X									
U/A and Culture	X									
HB₃Ag, HTLV III	X									
Brain CT or MRI	X									
Assess for adverse events status										X
PCR on PBL to detect NeoR gene	X	X	X	X				X		X
Tumor biopsy (if feasible)	X	X		X				X		X
Western blot (4070A envelope)	X									X
Serum assay for TNF	X	X	X	X	X	X		X		X

[1]To include assessment of *all* sites of disease.
[2]Includes total bilirubin, SGOT, LDH, Alkaline Phosphatase, Creatinine, Bun, CPK.

1. *Pretreatment*
   a. Complete physical examination, noting in detail the exact size and location of any lesions that exist
   b. Complete chemistry survey including electrolytes, liver function tests, calcium, magnesium, creatinine, BUN, CPK
   c. CBC differential count, PT, PTT, platelet count
   d. Urine analysis and culture
   e. Hepatitis screen
   f. HIV titer
   g. Pregnancy test if woman between the ages of 16 and 50
   h. Chest X ray
   i. Electrocardiogram
   j. Baseline X rays and nuclear medicine scans to evaluate the status of disease
   k. CT scan or MRI scan of brain
   l. 45 ml of clotted blood for serum storage and 45 ml of anticoagulate blood for mononuclear cell cryopreservation. Selected patients may undergo pretreatment lymphocytapheresis.
   m. Biopsy of tumor, if possible with minimal morbidity.

2. *During Treatment.* Patients will have a complete blood count and chemistry analysis panel at least every other day and a chest X ray performed each week during treatment.

During the infusion of the lymphocytes, patients will be monitored closely in the Surgical Intensive Care Unit. Vital signs including blood pressure, pulse, and respirations will be measured every 15 minutes during the cell infusion and every 30 minutes for at least four hours or until the patient is stable. A pulse oximeter will be used for on-line measurement of oxygen saturation during and for the four hours after cell infusion as well. If the systolic blood pressure drops below 80 mm/Hg, or the oxygen saturation drops below 90% during the cell infusion, the cell infusion will be terminated immediately.

3. *Post-Treatment.* Complete evaluation of evaluable lesions with physical examination, biopsy, if feasible, and appropriate X rays and/or scans prior to each cell infusion cycle and at approximately eight weeks after the end of treatment to evaluate response to treatment.

Western blot analysis of patient serum to determine possible exposure to retrovirus envelope proteins will be performed at 7 to 8 weeks after treatment.

4. *Criteria for Response. Complete response* is defined as the disappearance of all clinical evidence of disease for at least four weeks. *Partial response* is defined as the 50% or greater decrease of the sum of the products of perpendicular diameters of all lesions lasting at least four weeks with no increase in existing lesions or appearance of new lesions. Any patient having less than a partial response is considered to be non-responsive to treatment.

VI. Potential Side Effects and Reporting of Adverse Reactions

1. Adverse drug reaction reporting will be performed in accord with NCI current reporting requirements for Phase I studies as follows:

Report by telephone to IDB within 24 hours (301-496-7957, available 24 hours).

    a. All life-threatening events (Grade 4) which may be due to drug administration.

    b. All fatal events.

    c. The first occurrence of any *previously unknown* clinical event (regardless of Grade).

Written report to following within 10 working days to:

Investigational Drug Branch

P.O. Box 30012

Bethesda, Maryland 20824

2. Data will be submitted to CTMS at least once every two weeks. The NCI/DCT Case Report of ACES will be used to report to CTMS. All adverse reactions should also be reported to the IRB.

3. *Side Effects of IL-2.* A variety of side effects have been associated with IL-2 administration. We have had experience with the use of high-dose IL-2 either alone or in combination with cells or other cytokines in 1,039 courses in 652 patients.

TNF side effects including fever, chills, hypotension, oliguria, weight loss, nausea, vomiting, and malaise.

All side effects will be graded using the standard toxicity sheet used in all prior IL-2 related protocols.

4. *Potential Risks from Injection of Live Tumor.* These patients will receive the injection of approximately 0.1 gram of tumor into the skin or subcutaneous tissue of the anterior thigh. It should be emphasized that patients in this protocol will have histologically confirmed cancer with estimated tumor burdens of at least 10 grams or greater, which is 50 times the amount of the tumor cells used for these immunizations. Based on our experimental data it is unlikely that these gene-modified tumor cells will grow. These sites will be carefully monitored, however, and if tumor growth does occur, then this site has been selected so that it could be widely excised with minimum morbidity. A small chance does exist, however, that if this site does grow that it might lead to spread of the injected tumor cells to draining lymph nodes or other sites in the body. The patients included in this protocol, however, will have metastatic cancer with limited life expectancy. The spread of the injected tumor is considered unlikely and in this patient population is unlikely to negatively influence the prognosis from their disease.

If the gene-modified tumor cells do grow and produce TNF, then patients will be exposed to this systemic TNF. The maximum amount the TNF produced by the transduced tumor lines is about 15 ng$/10^6$ cells$/24$ hrs. If the tumors grow at all then they will be allowed to grow to a maximum of about 2×10^9 cells (or a 2 cm nodule) before they are excised. 2×10^9 cells will make about 30 ug of TNF for 24 hours. We and others have previously shown that 70 kg patients can tolerate approximately 600 µg TNF iv every 24 hours (8–10 µg/kg). Thus for a 70 kg human, the amount of TNF being produced by these gene-modified cells would be about 1/50th the amount of TNF already shown to be well tolerated by patients. It should be emphasized, however, that it is not expected that these tumor cells will grow based on experimental animal models. Further, if patients do develop signs of toxicity due to TNF exposure, then it will be possible to excise the local nodules in the anterior thigh. If tumor spreads from the local site, however, it may not be possible to remove all of the TNF-producing tumor.

5. *Risk from Murine Retrovirus.* Exposure of the cancer patient to retrovirus could theoretically pose a risk of insertional mutagenesis. It should be emphasized, however, that careful tests will be conducted to assure that the patient is not exposed to replication competent virus. The retrovirus derived from the Maloney murine leukemia virus has been modified so that it no longer contains any intact viral genes and thus cannot produce the envelope proteins necessary to package its RNA into an intact infectious virus (36,37,41,43,44). To assemble the retrovirus, a retrovirus packaging cell line was used that contained a second defective retrovirus which expresses the viral structural proteins. This packaging cell line does not produce replication competent retrovirus because of multiple modifications made to the second retrovirus that prevent its replication, including removal of signals required for RNA encapsidation, reverse transcription, and integration (37). Multiple assays will be performed on the final producer cell line, the retroviral vector supernatant as well as on the TIL prior to infusion to insure that no replication competent virus is present. These tests will include S + /L − assays including 3T3 amplification, PCR assays for the envelope gene, and assays for reverse transcriptase (42,43). Any supernatants or TIL with evidence of any replication competent virus will not be utilized. The 3T3 amplification and S + /L − assays are thought to be capable of detecting a single replication competent viral particle per ml (41).

Prior safety studies have shown that exposure of primates to large infusions of infectious murine amphotrophic virus produce no acute pathologic effects (44). In a study of 21 primates receiving retroviral mediated gene-modified autologous bone marrow cells, no animal showed evidence of toxicity related to the gene transfer as long as 5 years after infusion (45, unpublished data).

It should be emphasized, however, that tumor will be transduced with the retroviral vector supernatant and then the tumor will be washed extensively and then grown for several weeks in the absence of supernatant. The tumor will then be washed extensively again prior to reinfusion into the patient and patients will thus not be exposed directly to the retroviral vector.

VII. Statistical Considerations

Up to 14 patients with each type of cancer will be treated. If no responses are seen in these first 14 patients, no further patients with that histologic type of cancer will be admitted to the protocol.

MEDICAL RECORD
CONSENT TO PARTICIPATE IN A
CLINICAL RESEARCH STUDY
• **Adult Patient or** • **Parent, for Minor Patient**

INSTITUTE: NATIONAL CANCER INSTITUTE
STUDY NUMBER _____

PRINCIPAL INVESTIGATOR:
Steven A. Rosenberg, M.D., Ph.D.
STUDY TITLE: IMMUNIZATION OF CANCER PATIENTS USING AUTOLOGOUS CANCER CELLS MODIFIED BY INSERTION OF THE GENE FOR TUMOR NECROSIS FACTOR

INTRODUCTION

We invite you (or your child) to take part in a research study at the National Institutes of Health. It is important that you read and understand several general principles that apply to all who take part in our studies: (a) taking part in the study is entirely voluntary; (b) personal benefit may not result from taking part in the study, but knowledge may be gained that will benefit others; (c) you may withdraw from the study at any time without penalty or loss of any benefits to which you are otherwise entitled. The nature of the study, the risks, inconveniences, discomforts, and other pertinent information about the study are discussed below. You are urged to discuss any questions you have about this study with the staff members who explain it to you.

Nature of Study

The spread of your disease makes ineffective such standard therapies as drugs, surgery, and radiation. We are attempting to develop a procedure that may help fight your type of cancer. The procedure that we are offering you is highly experimental. The purpose of the study is to attempt to immunize you against your own cancer. It involves immunotherapy, using the body's immune system to treat the cancer. In laboratory studies in mice, we have shown that tumors that have had the gene for a substance called tumor necrosis factor (TNF) inserted are more readily recognized as foreign by the immune system of the mouse and are rejected. These gene-modified tumor cells can be used to immunize mice against their own cancers.

Earlier, when your tumor was surgically removed, we grew a sample of it in the laboratory in tissue culture. We inserted the gene for TNF into the cells of the tumor. The gene caused the cells of your tumor to produce TNF. We propose to inject these gene-modified tumor cells in three sites in your thigh, either in the skin or just below the skin. About three weeks later we will remove the lymph nodes that drain the tumor-bearing area and use them to grow immune cells called lymphocytes, which will later be given back to you as part of your immunotherapy. We will carefully observe the site of the tumor injection. If the tumor grows, we will remove it, attempt to grow immune lymphocytes from it, and if successful, use them in your treatment. If no tumor grows, the site will be surgically excised at about eight weeks after the injection. If we return lymphocytes to you for your treatment, you will also receive interleukin-2 (IL-2), a protein normally made by the body's immune system that can help the immune cells destroy your tumor. We cannot predict whether this approach will be of benefit to you in any way. It is a highly experimental technique. We are attempting to learn if it is of benefit in the treatment of patients with cancer.

Procedures

Before receiving any drug therapy you will have a number of tests to make sure you qualify for the study. The tests will be done on an in-patient or out-patient basis and may include the following: (1) X rays of the brain, chest, and abdomen; (2) blood tests; (3) testing your blood for the antibodies to human immunodeficiency virus (HIV), the virus that causes AIDS. If you are found to have these antibodies, you may not participate in this study. If you do qualify, you will undergo a series of procedures as part of the treatment.

The first step will be the injection of the gene-modified tissue-cultured tumor into three sites in your thigh. The tumor cells will be injected either into the skin or underneath the skin at three separate sites. The injections will be done with a standard needle and syringe and will be marked with tattooed dots. We will observe these sites carefully and have them inspected at least once a week.

If any tumor grows at these sites, we will allow it to grow until it reaches a size of about one-half inch. The site where the tumor was injected in the thigh will be surgically removed. The operation will probably be done under local anesthesia but may require general anesthesia. An incision several inches long will be necessary to do this and this can lead to bleeding, infection, and possibly swelling in the leg. Lymphocytes will be grown from any tumor found. It is possible that we will not be able to grow lymphocytes from this tumor deposit. The best chance for growing lymphocytes is in media already partly used by lymphocytes. We will make this media using lymphocytes taken from your vein blood by a procedure called apheresis. The lymphocytes are removed by a machine to which you are connected with two venous catheters (thin plastic tubes); the liquid part of the blood (plasma) and the red blood cells are returned to your veins. The procedure typically takes a few hours and rarely has any side effects.

If by three weeks no tumor has grown at the site of the injection, we will make a small incision into the groin and remove several lymph nodes from this area. This can usually be done under local anesthesia. We will attempt to grow these lymphocytes in culture for use in your treatment although it is possible that they will not grow.

If the lymphocytes from either the tumor site or from the draining lymph nodes do grow sufficiently, they will be transfused back into you along with IL-2, a protein normally made by the body's immune system. You will receive the IL-2 every eight hours until the maximum safe amount has been given. After approximately one week of recovery, a repeat treatment will be given using cells left over from the first week of treatment (if available) and more IL-2. It should be emphasized that the IL-2, the gene-modified tumor cells, and the TIL are all investigational agents. Approximately five weeks after that the effects of the treatment on your tumor will be measured by examination and X rays. The treatment may be repeated if frozen lymphocytes are available or additional sites of tumor can be removed and new lymphocytes grown. To give you the cells and IL-2 we will place a catheter in a vein in your upper chest wall or your neck. This catheter will be used to give the lymphocytes and can remain in place for the duration of your therapy. Placement of these catheters may be performed in the Surgical Intensive Care Unit. It is remotely possible that we might cause a small hole in the lung as we insert the catheter. This may require putting a tube in the chest for several days. The catheter may become infected. Appropriate treatment will be given if this occurs

Interleukin-2

Interleukin-2 can cause side effects that include weight gain due to retention of as much as 20 lbs of fluid over the course of a week. The weight gain can cause your arms and legs to swell and fluid to accumulate in the lungs. This can cause shortness of breath and may require placement of a tube in your windpipe (trachea) to allow mechanical breathing (breathing assisted by a machine). This would require transfer to the Surgical Intensive Care Unit. Less serious shortness of breath is common, and you may require oxygen delivered by a face mask during some portion of this treatment. Other side effects include fever and chills, which generally can be eliminated by appropriate medication. You also might develop nausea, diarrhea, a skin reaction with itching, nasal congestion, and abnormalities in kidney and liver function. Mental changes ranging from confusion and forgetfulness to disorientation have occasionally been observed. Other possible side effects include fatigue and mouth dryness. Your blood counts may drop to the point where you need red blood cell or platelet transfusions. Heart problems can occur, including irregular heart beat, low blood pressure, and heart attack. Some patients have developed a hole in their colon, resulting in abdominal inflammation and infection that required correction by surgery. In previous studies many of these side effects such as the weight gain, nausea, diarrhea, and liver and kidney dysfunction disappeared or were alleviated after stopping the IL-2 administration. Other unknown side effects may occur. It is very unlikely, though possible, that this treatment could kill you.

Immune Lymphocytes

The administration of the lymphocytes may cause fever, chills, and shortness or breath. Based on our previous experience, these side effects are expected and should only last a few hours. Because these lymphocytes are grown from your tumor, it is possible that the lymphocytes returned to you may contain tumor cells. This may make your condition worse. We will carefully examine the lymphocytes that you are to be given to decrease the chance of this occurrence.

Although administration of immune lymphocytes can shrink tumors in some patients, many patients do not respond to the procedure and even those that exhibit shrinkage may show regrowth of the tumor after a short period of time (months).

Tumor Necrosis Factor

Recent scientific advances have made it possible to modify the genetic makeup of tumors so that they can stimulate a greater response by the immune system. The scientific advance is called "retroviral-mediated gene transfer" and allows us to insert a gene into some of your tumor cells, stimulating them to produce a hormone called tumor necrosis factor (TNF). This hormone is naturally produced in the body in small amounts. The cells we give you may, however, produce too much TNF throughout the body. TNF is thought to play a role in body defenses against cancer. Giving too much TNF may be dangerous and may cause life-threatening low blood pressure. TNF can also cause fever, chills, low urine output, weight loss, nausea, vomiting, and fatigue. We have inserted into your tumor, by a special laboratory technique, not only the human gene for TNF but a second gene taken from a bacterium that causes the tumor cells to be resistant to an antibiotic, neomycin. A gene is a part of a chromosome (hereditary material) that contains the information a cell needs to make proteins.

The following procedure was used to insert these genes into your tumor. The tumor cells were attached to mouse virus genetic material that has the capacity to act as a carrier of foreign genes from one cell to another, taking the two genes with it. These tumor cells are then grown in the laboratory in large numbers. Special tests are performed on these cells to determine that they contain the new genes and that TNF is being produced.

There are some potential risks to this procedure. First, even though the mouse virus used to insert the gene into your lymphocytes cannot grow and is considered harmless to you, it is possible that events could occur within the cell that allow the virus to grow. To minimize this possibility, the gene-marked tumor cells will be tested and if any virus is found, the cells will be discarded. Second, the inserted gene produces a protein that inactivates certain antibiotics. These antibiotics are not commonly used to treat infections in humans, and many other antibiotics are available that will not be inactivated and would be effective in treating bacterial infections. We emphasize that this procedure, called retroviral-mediated gene transfer, has been used before only in very few human patients. Because this procedure is relatively new, it is possible that despite our extensive efforts, other unforeseen problems may occur, including the very remote possibility of death.

You will undergo biopsy of tumor and other tissue, if available, on several occasions before and after the tumor infiltrating lymphocytes (TIL) from either the tumor or local lymph nodes are given. A maximum of five biopsies of lesions in or under the skin may be performed. The biopsies are done under local anesthesia and are associated with minor discomfort lasting about 24 hours. Blood and tissue specimens will be taken where possible to follow the life span and function of the marked cells.

This clinical procedure has attracted a great deal of attention from the lay media. We will make every effort to protect the confidentiality of you and your family. However, because of this media interest there is a greater risk than usual that information concerning you and your treatment will appear publicly without your consent. A qualified representative of the manufacturer of IL-2 may have access to the patient and study records on this protocol.

The injection of live tumor cells back into you is unusual and highly experimental. Although any tumor appearing in the thigh can likely be controlled by surgical removal (or possibly by adding radiation therapy), these measures could fail, resulting in progressive tumor in the thigh. It is also possible that this tumor may spread from this site and produce TNF at other sites and that we may not be able to control this. We do emphasize, however, that the amount of tumor that we are injecting into you is less than 1/50th of the total amount of tumor we estimate is already in your body. It is, however, possible that you may suffer injury or disability such as pain, bleeding, or infection from the tumor injected into the skin of the thigh.

Possible Benefits for Participants

We cannot predict whether this new procedure will be of benefit to you. In past lymphocyte transfer studies, some tumor shrinkage was observed in some individuals but not in others. Even those tumors that exhibit shrinkage may show regrowth of the tumor after a short period of time (months). At this stage in your illness, tumor shrinkage may be associated with prolongation of life.

Alternative Treatments

There are no known curative treatments for patients with your disease. You could also consider receiving other experimental treatments such as experimental chemotherapy. The option also exists to receive no treatment at this time.

Follow Up

After you receive each cycle of this procedure, you will be discharged from the hospital. At about five weeks after the last treatment you will be required to return to the NIH for follow-up studies. Tests used to decide if your tumor has responded to the procedure will be similar to those you had before beginning the therapy.

When you have completed your participation in this study, you will be eligible to be considered for participation in other research protocols at the National Cancer Institute and you will receive care as indicated by your disease or you will be referred elsewhere for care.

As this is a new procedure, side effects that may cause your condition to deteriorate may be encountered. You will be watched closely for any side effects.

You are free to withdraw your consent to participate in this study at the National Cancer Institute and seek care from any physician at any time. If you withdraw from the study after the injection of the gene-modified tumor cells but before the surgical excision of the injection site, then we would be willing to immediately resect the injection site or observe the injection site at monthly intervals and resect the site if tumor appears.

If you have any questions concerning issue of patients' rights, you can contact *Ms. Betty Schwering,* phone *#(301) 496-2626,* in the Clinical Center, NIH.

MEDICAL RECORD
INCLUSION OF HIV TESTING IN CONSENT
TO PARTICIPATE IN A
CLINICAL RESEARCH STUDY

As part of your participation in this study, it will be necessary to test your blood for the presence of antibodies to the Human Immunodeficiency Virus (HIV), the virus that causes Acquired Immune Deficiency Syndrome (AIDS). In order to perform the test, a small amount of blood (approximately 2 teaspoons) will be withdrawn from one of your arms with a needle. You may experience some slight discomfort at the needle entry site and there may be some bruising. In addition, there is a very small risk of your fainting or of infection at the needle entry site. If your test results are found to be positive, or if you are otherwise diagnosed as having AIDS, you should be aware of the following Clinical Center HIV Testing Policy:

1. You physician will notify you promptly of the HIV test results.

2. Your physician and/or the Clinical Center HIV counselor will offer you, and any current and/or ongoing sexual partner(s) (spouses are generally considered to be current or ongoing sexual partners) or needle-sharing partner(s) you identify, information on the meaning of the test results and how to prevent the spread of the infection.

3. Because the virus may be transmitted in several ways, it is important that you inform sexual and/or needle-sharing partner(s) that any, or all, of them may have been exposed to the HIV virus and encourage them to be tested. If you request it, staff at the Clinical Center will assist you in notifying your partner(s) and arrange counseling for them through an HIV counselor.

4. The results of your HIV test and/or documentation of the diagnosis of AIDS will become a part of your Clinical Center medical record and, as such, will be protected from unauthorized disclosure by the Federal Privacy Act of 1974. In general, access to your medical record will be restricted to those health care professionals directly involved in your care or in the conduct of ongoing biomedical research, and information is not usually released to other third parties without your permission or that of your designated representative. However, there are some particular routine uses of such information of which you should be aware.

   a. If you are unwilling or unable to notify your partner(s), the Clinical Center is responsible for attempting to contact and inform them of their possible exposure to the virus. Reasonable attempts will be made to protect your identity, including withholding your name when notifying any partner(s) of their possible exposure. Some notification or counseling of current and/or ongoing partners may be carried out through arrangements with, or referral to, local public health agencies.

   b. A summary of your care at the Clinical Center will be sent to the physician who referred you here for treatment.

   c. The Clinical Center may report certain communicable diseases, including AIDS, to appropriate State and Federal government agencies.

If you have any questions regarding the HIV testing or the information provided above, you are encouraged to discuss them with your physician and/or a Clinical Center HIV counselor (496-8955).

MEDICAL RECORD
CONSENT TO PARTICIPATE IN A
CLINICAL RESEARCH STUDY
• Adult Patient or   • Parent, for Minor Patient

STUDY NUMBER: _____

OTHER PERTINENT INFORMATION

1. **Confidentiality.** When results of a study such as this are reported in medical journals or at meetings, the identification of those taking part is withheld. Medical records of Clinical Center patients are maintained according to current requirements, and are made available for review, as required by the Food and Drug Administration or other authorized users, only under the guidelines established by the Federal Privacy Act.
2. **Policy Regarding Research-Related Injuries.** The Clinical Center will provide short-term medical care for any physical injury resulting from your participation in research here. Neither the Clinical Center nor the Federal government provide long-term medical care or financial compensation for such injuries, except as may be provided through whatever remedies are normally available under law.
3. **Payments.** If you are a patient, you are not paid for taking part in NIH studies. Exceptions for volunteers will be guided by Clinical Center policies.
4. **Problems or Questions.** Should any problem or question arise with regard to this study, with regard to your risk as a participant in clinical research, or with regard to any research-related injury, you should contact the principal investigator, Dr. Steven Rosenberg, or other staff members also involved in this study at Building 10, Room 2B42, National Institutes of Health, Bethesda, Maryland 20205. Telephone: (301) 496-4164.
5. **Consent Document.** It is suggested that you retain a copy of this document for your later reference and personal records.

COMPLETE APPROPRIATE ITEM BELOW, A OR B:

A. Adult Patient's Consent.
   I have read the explanation about this study and have been given the opportunity to discuss it and to ask questions. I hereby consent to take part in this study.

_____

Signature of Adult Patient & Date Signed

B. Parent's Permission for Minor Patient.
   I have read the explanation about this study and have been given the opportunity to discuss it and to ask questions. I hereby give permission for my child to take part in this study.
   (Attach NIH 2514-2, Minor's Assent, if applicable)

_____

Signature of Parent(s) & Date Signed

_____

(if other than parent, specify relationship)

_____

_____
Signature of Investigator & Date Signed

_____
Signature of Witness & Date Signed

ADDENDUM TO OPERATIVE CONSENT FORM

As a part of your operation, a cancer will be surgically removed. We will attempt to grow your cancer in the laboratory and establish a cultured cell line from your cancer. This cell line may be used to study the characteristics of your tumor and may be used in laboratory tests. It is possible that we will attempt to insert foreign genes into your tumor. It is unlikely, though possible, that we will be able to use this cultured cell line to test highly experimental treatment procedures. If you are offered any of these procedures, then we will seek your written informed consent explaining the procedures in detail before any treatments with this cell line are initiated.

_____
Patient's Signature

APPENDIX

S + /L − Assay. The cat fibroblast line PG-4 or mink lung line $MiCl_1$ is used as the indicator cell line. Twenty-four hours prior to virus exposure, cells are plated on 6 well dishes, 1×10^5 cells per well in 1 ml of medium. On the day of infection, 0.5 ml of DEAE Dextran (20 µg/ml in medium) is added to each well and incubated with cells for 30 minutes. Dextran is removed and 0.5 ml of test sample is added and incubated for 2 hours at 37°C. After 2 hours the test material is replaced with 2.5 ml of medium and incubated for 3 days. Foci of transformed cells are determined microscopically with a 10 × objective and the focus-forming units per ml (ffu/ml) calculated.

3T3 Amplification. 3T3 cells are maintained in Dulbecco's modified Eagle's medium with 10% fetal calf serum and 2 mM L-glutamine; the cells are grown at 37°C, in 5% CO_2. Cells are plated at 1×10^5 cells per well in 6 well dishes twenty-four hours prior to sample exposure. Medium is removed and 0.5 ml of supernate samples are added per well; polybrene (8 µg/ml) is used to enhance viral infection. Cocultivation with cells is performed overnight in a volume of 1 ml with polybrene (8 µg/ml). After infection the samples are removed and 2.5 ml fresh medium is added. Cells are split 1:10 when confluent and carried for 3 weeks. At the end of the first and third week, when plates are confluent, fresh medium is added to the well and collected 20 hours later for analysis in the S + /L − assay.

Polymerase Chain Reaction. DNA is isolated from both uninfected and transduced TIL cells using standard techniques and subjected to polymerase chain reaction. In this assay $1 - 5$ µg of DNA is added to a 0.5 ml microcentrifuge tube containing 100 µl of 50 mM KCL, 10 mM Tris-HCl (pH = 8.3), 1.5 mM $MgCl_2$, 0.01% gelatin, 200 µM each deoxynucleotide triphosphate, 1.0 µM envelope primer 1, 1.0 µM envelope primer 2, and 2.5 U of Taq DNA polymerase. All reagents, with the exception of TIL cell DNA and the envelope primers, are supplied in kits purchased from Perkin Elmer Cetus (GeneAmp kit). The samples are then placed in a DNA Thermal Cycler instrument (Perkin Elmer Cetus) and subjected to 30 cycles of 3 minutes each of 94°C denaturation, 53°C annealing, and 72°C polymerization conditions. At the completion of the cycling, the amplified DNA sample is removed and analyzed by agarose gel electrophoresis followed by Southern blot analysis using a radiolabeled DNA probe isolated from the envelope gene of the amphotropic virus 4070A. Final analysis for the presence of amphotropic envelope sequences is obtained by autoradiography of the Southern blot.

CLINICAL CENTER HOSPITAL IMPACT STATEMENT
PROJECTED UTILIZATION OF RESOURCES

Protocol Title: Immunization of Cancer Patients Using Autologous Cancer Cells Modified by Insertion of the Gene for Tumor Necrosis Factor

Institute: NCI

Principal Investigator: Steven A. Rosenberg, M.D., Ph.D.

Start Date for Study: 4/1/91

Duration of Study: 3 yrs

Drug Trial: Yes ( ) No ( )

Phase: I (x) II ( ) III ( )

IND or IDE Required: Yes (x) No ( )

Radiation Safety Review Required: Yes ( ) No (xx)

Total Number (#) of Patients in Study: __50__ pts.

patients in first year: __29__ pts.

maximum # patients at any time: __1__ pts. per __week__

Number of Inpatient Admissions per Patient: __3__ adm. pt.

admissions in first year: __3__ adm. pt.

admissions in each subsequent year: __0__ adms. pt.

Average Length of Stay per Admission: __7__ days adm.

length of first admission: __7__ days adm.

length of each follow-up admission: __7__ days adm.

Number of Surgical Procedures per Patient: __1__ procedures/patient

length of pre-op stay: __1__ days

length of post-op stay: __2__ days

Nursing Unit(s): __2East, 2J__

Clinic Floor: __3rd floor__

Special Care Units: (Check any that will be used during the study)
2J (x)   10D ( )   12W-LAF ( )   5W-Care Room ( )   Other: _____

Level of Nursing Care: (Check the most intensive level expected)

( ) Ambulatory Care: e.g., 0–3 hrs. per 24 hrs.
( ) Minimal Care (mild symptoms; minimal assistance): e.g., 3–6 hrs. per 24 hrs.
( ) Moderate Care (frequent treatment, observation or instruction): e.g., 6–12 hrs. per 24 hrs.
( ) Complex Care (extreme symptoms, need full assistance): e.g., 12–24 hrs. per 24 hrs.

	# Visits in first	# Visits each subsequent
Total Outpatient Visits per Patient: __3__ visits pt.	year: __3__ visits pt.	year: __3__ visits pt.

Is a flowchart or scheme included in the protocol? Yes ( ) No ( ). Please include a scheme or flowchart for complex protocols.

Additional Comments:

PROTOCOL IMPLEMENTATION PLANNING DOCUMENT

DATE: March 19, 1991   **ANALYSIS BY:** Vera Wheeler, RN
                                 PHONE EXT./BEEPER:

PROTOCOL TITLE: Immunization of Cancer Patients Using Autologous
                   Cancer Cells Modified by Insertion of the Gene for
                   Tumor Necrosis Factor

PROTOCOL NUMBER: **P.I.:** Steven A. Rosenberg, MD, PhD
                             PHONE EXT./BEEPER:

INSTITUTE(S): National Cancer Institute, Surgery Branch

PROPOSED START DATE: April 1, 1991

Protocol Summary. Patient Population: Any cancer patient with advanced disease, 6 months life expectancy or less, and who has failed standard treatment options.
    Number of Patients: 50 pts. over 3 years.
    Nursing Units Involved: SICU/2 East/OP3
    Tumor tissue cultures will be established for patients having surgical resection of their malignancy as part of their treatment course. The gene coding for IL-2 will be introduced into the cultured tumor cells. The gene-altered tumor cells will then be injected subcutaneously and intradermally into the thigh of the patient (less than 1/50th of the patient's total tumor burden). The tumor implant site will be closely observed for growth as well as the impact of these gene-altered tumor cells on other established metastatic tumor sites. When the implanted tumor reaches 1–2 cm. size, it will be removed and grown using standard TIL culture procedures. At three weeks post-tumor implant, the patient will undergo resection of several lymph nodes from the draining superficial inguinal area near the tumor implant

site. Attempts will be made to grow these lymphocytes and the above TIL for adoptive cellular therapy, to be reinfused in the patient with IL-2 as described in previous protocols.

Nursing Impact Analysis. This protocol appears to build on two Surgery Branch protocols which have just begun, i.e., Dr. Rosenberg's gene therapy protocol for TIL modified with the TNF gene and Dr. Yang's subcutaneous tumor implant for generation of TIL. It is yet unclear how these two studies will impact nursing, and therefore it is hard to predict the nursing impact of this initial research proposal at this time. For example, it is unknown at present what side effect the patient will experience as a result of TIL with the TNF gene, how long these side effects will last, and if there is any long-term sequelae. There is no experience at present with the IL-2 gene inserted into TIL.

There will be some increase in the number of surgical procedures of a minor nature: Resection of the draining lymph nodes at three weeks, resection of the implanted tumor for TILS or resection of the implant site at three weeks if the tumor doesn't grow. Presumably, the initial tumor culture will be obtained from patients already scheduled for a surgical procedure.

PATIENT/FAMILY TEACHING: _X_ ROUTINE___ EXTENSIVE
Materials presently exist for teaching patients about IL-2 effects, TIL therapy, and other aspects of treatment. It would be helpful to develop materials on the tumor-immunization procedure and TNF.

NURSING EDUCATION

PROTOCOL RELATED: The nursing units for this study are well acquainted with the proposed therapeutic agents of TIL and IL-2 administration. The current protocols for subcutaneous implanted tumor and gene therapy will assist in the implementation of this proposed study as nursing staff will become acquainted with how tumor immunization is managed. It will, however, be helpful to have the P. I. introduce this protocol to the combined nursing staff prior to the first patient in order to answer questions about the study's purpose, safety, and nursing responsibilities.

POPULATION: Unchanged.

TECHNOLOGY/PROCEDURE RELATED: No special equipment required.

INVESTIGATIONAL AGENTS/PHARMACOKINETICS: Lymphocytes derived from resected lymph nodes are a new form of cellular adoptive therapy; however, they will be administered in the same manner as TIL.

Patient Stay.
_____ LOS <24 HRS; 1 OP VISIT/MONTH
_____ LOS 24 HRS to 1 WEEK; OP VISITS EVERY 1–4 WEEKS

__X__ LOS > 4 WEEKS; SPECIAL CARE > 5 DAYS; OP VISITS EVERY
          2–3 DAYS; OP VISITS EVENINGS OR WEEKENDS.
COMMENT: Patients will potentially require a special care unit for five days
or greater.

ETHICAL/LEGAL/CULTURAL: The consent document provides an explanation of the risks of the tumor implant procedure, the potential toxicities of
administration of immune lymphocytes and of IL-2.

SUPPLIES/EQUIPMENT:
__X__ EQUIPMENT ROUTINELY AVAILABLE
_____ INCREASED VOLUME:

_____ SPECIAL EQUIPMENT AND SUPPLIES REQUIRED AS FOL-
LOWS:

Inter-Unit/Service/Hospital Coordination.
Inpatient/Outpatient Clinics: No change expected in the current level of coordi-
nation between OP3 and the inpatient units. There may be an occasional emer-
gency admit for immunotherapy patients requiring prompt medical intervention.
This is the present situation and it is as yet unknown whether these protocol
patients will have more emergent problems.
Inpatient/Inpatient Areas. No change from the current level of transfers.
On-Pass Patients. No impact.
Out-of-Hospital Transfers/Transportation. No needs identified.
Environment/Milieu. No needs identified.

Clinical Center Departments.

ANESTHESIA	X NO IMPACT	___ OTHER:
AUDIOLOGY	X NO IMPACT	___ OTHER:
BIOETHICS	X NO IMPACT	___ OTHER:
BIOMEDICAL ENGINEERING	X NO IMPACT	___ OTHER:
BLOOD BANK	X NO IMPACT	___ OTHER:
CHILD HEALTH WORKER	X NO IMPACT	___ OTHER:
CLINICAL PATHOLOGY	___ NO IMPACT	X OTHER:

Dr. Galnick's service: CBC with diff QOD.

CONSULT MEDICAL SERVICES	X NO IMPACT	___ OTHER:
CRITICAL CARE MED	X NO IMPACT	___ OTHER:
EPIDEMIOLOGY	X NO IMPACT	___ OTHER:
MESSENGER & ESCORT/VOLUNTEERS	X NO IMPACT	___ OTHER:
MIS	X NO IMPACT	___ OTHER:
NUCLEAR MEDICINE	___ NO IMPACT	X OTHER:

Pretreatment and Post-treatment nuclear med scans to evaluate the status of
disease.

NUTRITION	___ NO IMPACT	X OTHER:
PHARMACY	X NO IMPACT	___ OTHER:
POLICE	X NO IMPACT	___ OTHER:

RADIATION ONCOLOGY	X NO IMPACT	___ OTHER:
RADIOLOGY	X NO IMPACT	___ OTHER:
RECREATIONAL THERAPY	X NO IMPACT	___ OTHER:
REHABILITATION MED	X NO IMPACT	___ OTHER:
RESPIRATORY THERAPY	X NO IMPACT	___ OTHER:
SCHOOL	X NO IMPACT	___ OTHER:
SOCIAL WORKER	X NO IMPACT	___ OTHER:

Outstanding Concerns/Questions to Be Answered.

It would be helpful to see final version of protocol prior to implementation to identify any late changes which may impact on nursing care of these patients.

PART III

THE TEN MOST COMMON CANCERS

Introduction

ᴘᴀʀᴛ III ɪs ᴀ ʀᴇᴠɪᴇᴡ ᴏғ ᴡʜᴀᴛ ᴀʀᴇ ɴᴏᴡ ᴛʜᴇ ᴛᴇɴ ᴍᴏsᴛ ᴄᴏᴍᴍᴏɴ cancers in the United States, in order of incidence: lung, colon and rectum, breast, prostate, bladder, non-Hodgkin's lymphoma, uterus, oral cavity (including lip and pharynx), pancreas, and leukemia. For each we describe symptoms, screening, diagnosis, laboratory tests, and stages, and present charts listing the status, incidence, mortality, known or possible causes, preventive lifestyle changes, medical intervention, and, where there is significant new work, research frontiers.

In 1990, approximately 1,040,000 new cases of cancer were diagnosed in the United States (not including nonmelanoma skin cancer), and 510,000 people died from cancer. Although the five-year survival rate has varied greatly—it is currently 3 percent for pancreatic cancer and 88 percent for testicular cancer—since 1960 it has improved for both white and black patients. In 1960, it was 39 percent for white and 27 percent for black patients; in 1970, it was 43 percent and 31 percent, respectively; in 1980, it was 51 percent and 38 percent, respectively. The overall five-year survival rate in 1990 was 52 percent (National Cancer Institute and American Cancer Society).

Each chapter in this section includes information about the twenty-four-hour Cancer Hotline and fax service established by the National Cancer Institute. These are gold mines of timely information that all cancer patients and their families should know about.

Chapter 9

Lung Cancer

LUNG CANCER IS THE MOST COMMON FATAL CANCER IN THE UNITED States. It is the most common cancer of men and, since 1955, has increased dramatically in women, even those who do not smoke. In many industrial countries, lung cancer is now responsible for approximately 40 percent of all cancer deaths in men and 30 percent in women. There is a higher incidence of lung cancer among black men than white men; women show no differences by race. In black men lung cancer is, after coronary heart disease, the second most common cause of death. National surveys since 1914 have shown that more black men than white men smoke, and they often choose cigarettes with higher tar content (Henderson et al. 1991, p. 1,131).

Although 85 percent of all lung cancers are thought to be caused by smoking, some do occur among nonsmokers, perhaps due to second-hand smoke. Because it is highly malignant, the earlier lung cancer is diagnosed, the better the chances of cure, especially for certain types. There are two types of lung cancer: small-cell and non-small-cell. The cancer cells of each type grow and spread in different ways, and they are treated differently. Non-small-cell lung cancer is usually associated with prior smoking, passive smoking, or radon exposure. The three main kinds of non-small-cell lung cancer are named for the type of cells found in them: squamous-cell (the flat cells that line the lung passage) carcinoma (also called epidermoid carcinoma), adenocarcinoma (in cells that form glandlike tumors), and large-cell carcinoma. Non-small-cell lung cancer is a common disease usually treated by surgical removal or radiation therapy, which uses high-dose X rays to kill the cancer cells. The prognosis and treatment depend on the stage of the cancer (whether it is just in the lung or has spread to other places), the type of lung cancer, and the patient's general health.

Small-cell lung cancer is a disease in which cancer cells are found in the tissues of the lungs. Small-cell lung cancer is sometimes called oat-cell lung cancer, because the cells are small (half to three-quarters the size of cells in non-small-cell carcinoma) and round. Small-cell lung cancer is usually found in cigarette smokers or former cigarette smokers. Like most cancer, small-cell lung cancer is best treated when it is diagnosed early. The following list explains screening, diagnosis, and examinations.

Screening

Periodic chest X rays, even in smokers, have not proved useful in screening for lung cancer.

Diagnosis

Symptoms
   Most common symptom is a wheezing "smoker's cough" that persists for months or even years.
   Increased, sometimes blood-streaked, sputum.
   Persistent ache in the chest.
Physical Examination
   Evidence of congestion (fluid in air spaces) of the lung.
   Collection of fluid in space between lung and chest wall, called the pleura.
   Enlarged lymph nodes in the neck indicating metastasis.
Routine Laboratory Tests
   Blood tests for general health status (anemia, infections, blood-clotting capacity).
   Urine analysis to determine kidney function.
   Liver function tests to determine whether cancer has spread to liver.
   Electrocardiogram to evaluate heart function.
   Chest X ray to visualize cancer, enlarged lymph nodes, pneumonia, or fluid accumulation.

Special Laboratory Tests   To diagnose the specific type of cancer and to "stage" it—that is, to determine whether it has spread to other organs such as the brain, bone, or liver.

SPUTUM EXAMINATION   To check for cancer cells.

BRONCHOSCOPY   With a special instrument called a broncho-scope, the physician can take cells from the walls of the bronchial tubes or cut out small pieces of tissue (called a biopsy) and examine them under a microscope to determine whether there are any cancer cells.

THORACENTESIS AND ASPIRATION BIOPSY   A cut is made in the skin and a needle inserted between the ribs to draw out (aspirate) any fluid that has collected in the pleural space (thoracentesis) or fragments of cancer tissue (aspiration biopsy).

METASTATIC WORKUP   Sometimes performed to stage the cancer and includes radionuclide "scans" of the brain, liver, and bone using radioactive materials that localize in cancer tissues and show up on X rays. Also included may be a needle aspiration of bone marrow in sternum or hip to look for cancer cells.

CT SCAN OR MRI IMAGING   These tests—computerized tomography and magnetic resonance imaging—are done to clearly define the location and size of a tumor as well as to check for metastasis.

THORACOTOMY   If biopsy of lung tumor cannot be obtained by the methods already described, this exploratory chest operation will be performed. Thoracotomy is major surgery and will be done only after the metastatic workup has been performed and other tests have not located and identified the type of cancer. The chest is opened surgically and the tumor located and biopsied.

Although not all of these tests are required for each patient, enough of them must be performed to obtain a specific diagnosis upon which all future therapy will be based.

Stages of Non-Small-Cell Lung Cancer

As explained, once lung cancer has been diagnosed, a number of tests will be done to determine whether it has spread to other parts of the body. The physician needs to know the stage to plan treatment. The stages of non-small-cell lung cancer are named as follows:

OCCULT STAGE   Cancer cells are found in sputum, but no tumor can be found in the lung.

STAGE O	Cancer is found only in a local area and only in a few layers of cells. It has not grown through the top lining of the lung. Another term for this type of lung cancer is carcinoma *in situ*.
STAGE I	Cancer is only in the lung, and normal tissue is around it.
STAGE II	Cancer has spread to nearby lymph nodes.
STAGE III	Cancer has spread to the chest wall or diaphragm near the lung, to the lymph nodes in the area that separates the two lungs (mediastinum), or to the lymph nodes on the other side of the chest or in the neck. Stage III is further divided into stage IIIA (can be operated on) and stage IIIB (cannot be operated on).
STAGE IV	Cancer has spread to other parts of the body.
RECURRENT	Cancer has come back (recurred) after previous treatment.

Treatment of Non-Small-Cell Lung Cancer

Patients with non-small-cell lung cancer can be divided into three groups, depending on the stage of the cancer and the treatment that is planned. The first group includes patients whose cancers can be taken out by surgery. The operation that takes out only a small part of the lung is called a *wedge resection*. When a whole section (lobe) of the lung is taken out, the operation is called a *lobectomy*. When one whole lung is taken out, it is called a *pneumonectomy*.

Radiation therapy may be used to treat patients in this group who cannot have surgery because of other medical problems. Like surgery, radiation therapy is called *local* treatment because it works only on the cells in the area to be treated.

The second group of patients has lung cancer that has spread to nearby tissue or lymph nodes. These patients can be treated with radiation therapy alone or with surgery and radiation.

The third group of patients has lung cancer that has spread to other parts of the body. Radiation therapy may be used to shrink the cancer and to relieve pain.

Chemotherapy for non-small-cell lung cancer is being studied in many clinical trials.

TREATMENT BY STAGE

OCCULT STAGE	Tests are done to find the main tumor. Lung cancer that is found at this early stage can be cured by surgery.
STAGE 0	These very early cancers can be cured by surgery. However, these patients may get a second lung cancer that may not be able to be taken out by surgery.
STAGE I	Treatment choices are surgery or radiation therapy (for patients who cannot be operated on).
STAGE II	Treatment choices are surgery to take out the tumor and lymph nodes or radiation therapy (for patients who cannot be operated on).
STAGE IIIA	Treatment choices are surgery, radiation therapy, or both.
STAGE IIIB	These patients are not helped by surgery; radiation therapy alone is used to control the disease.
STAGE IV	These patients are treated with radiation therapy. Chemotherapy is being evaluated as a treatment option. They also need other kinds of care to control pain and other problems.
RECURRENT	When lung cancer comes back again (recurs), radiation therapy or chemotherapy can help to control pain.

Stages of Small-Cell Lung Cancer

Once small-cell lung cancer has been found, more tests will be done to find out whether cancer cells have spread from one or both lungs to other parts of the body. The stages of small-cell lung cancer are named as follows:

LIMITED STAGE	Cancer is found only in one lung and in nearby lymph nodes.
EXTENSIVE STAGE	Cancer has spread beyond the lung to other tissues in the chest or to other parts of the body.
RECURRENT STAGE	Cancer has come back after it has been treated. It may recur in the lungs or in another part of the body.

Treatment by Stage

The treatment for *limited stage* may be one of the following:

1. Chemotherapy and radiation therapy to the chest with or without radiation therapy to the brain to prevent spread of the cancer *(prophylactic cranial irradiation).*
2. Chemotherapy with or without prophylactic cranial irradiation.
3. Surgery followed by chemotherapy with or without prophylactic cranial irradiation.

Clinical trials are testing new drugs and new ways of administering all of the above treatments.

The treatment for *extensive stage* may be one of the following:

1. Chemotherapy with or without prophylactic cranial irradiation.
2. Chemotherapy and radiation therapy to the chest with or without prophylactic cranial irradiation.
3. Radiation therapy to places in the body where the cancer has spread, such as the bone or spine, to relieve symptoms.

Clinical trials are testing new drugs and new ways of administering all of the above treatments.

The treatment for *recurrent small-cell lung cancer* may be one of the following:

1. Radiation therapy to reduce discomfort.
2. A clinical trial testing new drugs.

To learn more about lung cancer, call the National Cancer Institute's Information Service at 1-800-4-CANCER. The Cancer Information Service can also send the following free booklets about lung cancer:

Research Report: Cancer of the Lung
What You Need to Know About Cancer

The following chart summarizes the current facts about lung cancer.

LUNG CANCER

STATUS	157,000 new cases in the United States during 1990
	Most common cancer
	Accounts for approximately 15% of all cancers diagnosed
	Predicted to be major health problem for decades to come
INCIDENCE	Increased approximately 30% between 1973 and 1987
MORTALITY	Leading cause of deaths from cancer
	Increased approximately 34% between 1973 and 1987
	Predicted to increase in women for 10 years; now leading cause of death for women, surpassing breast cancer
	Leveled off in men due to cessation of smoking
KNOWN CAUSE	Tobacco, especially cigarette smoking
LIFESTYLE CHANGES TO PREVENT THE CANCER	Stop smoking, even low-tar cigarettes
	Increase consumption of fruits and leafy vegetables that contain beta-carotene
	Increase consumption of foods containing vitamins C and E
MEDICAL INTERVENTION	Encourage lifestyle changes, to discontinue smoking, especially for women and all adolescents
	Encourage consumption of foods

containing beta-carotene and vitamins C and E

Advise the public about the risks of passive smoking

Routine assays for alterations in protooncogenes (c-*myc*, L-*myc*, N-*myc*, and H-*ras*) and tumor-suppressor genes (p53, Rb, and locus on chromosome 3)

RESEARCH FRONTIERS

The tumor-suppressor gene, p53, plays a crucial role in the origin of lung cancer; 50% of lung cancers and 100% of small-cell lung cancers have mutations in this gene.

The alterations in the DNA of the p53 gene are characteristic of those produced by mutagens in tobacco smoke.

Eventual genetic testing for alterations in the p53 gene will indicate which individuals are at increased risk for lung cancer.

Loss of function of p53 (an increase in p53 mutant protein) is under study as a marker for poor prognosis.

Studies are evaluating the presence of antibodies against p53 protein in patients' serum as a diagnostic and prognostic marker.

Abnormalities in chromosomes 3, 5, 13, and 17 occur in lung-cancer cells.

Sputum can be tested for cells with genetic changes that occur in lung cancer.

Chapter 10

Colon and Rectal Cancers

COLON AND RECTAL CANCERS ARE THE SECOND MOST COMMON CANcer in the United States (after lung cancer but excluding skin cancers), accounting for 15 percent of all cancers. In contrast to lung and, of course, breast cancer, they are found equally in men and women. Colon cancer increases remarkably with age; its incidence increases steadily between the ages of twenty and ninety. It occurs ten times more frequently in individuals over sixty-five than in those aged forty-five. When diagnosed early, cancers of the colon and rectum can often be cured. Therefore the public should be informed of the symptoms of these cancers and, if they appear, should see a physician immediately.

In cancer of the colon, cancer cells are found in the tissues of the colon. The colon is part of the body's digestive system. This system is made up of the esophagus, stomach, and the small and large intestines. The last six feet of intestine is called the large bowel or colon.

Screening

Like most cancers, cancer of the colon is best treated when it is diagnosed early. Because of this, screening tests (such as a rectal exam, proctoscopy, and colonoscopy) should be done on people who are at risk: those over age forty who have a family history of cancer of the colon, rectum, or female organs, or who have a history of ulcerative colitis (ulcers in the lining of the large intestines). The physician may order these tests to look for cancer if the patient has a change in bowel habits or any bleeding from the rectum.

Diagnosis

Symptoms   The patient with colon or rectal cancer will often experience a series of gastrointestinal (GI) symptoms and signs. The most critical sign, rectal bleeding, as indicated by red blood in stools or by black stools, should lead to an immediate appointment with a physician. Other manifestations are abdominal cramps, constipation alternating with diarrhea, loss of appetite, weight loss, weakness, and pallid complexion.

Physical Examination   After a complete physical examination, the physician will do a digital rectal examination in which, wearing a thin glove, he or she inserts a finger into the rectum and feels for lumps.

Routine Laboratory Tests   Routine blood tests may reveal an anemia due to internal bleeding from the tumor. A *guaiac test* may detect small amounts of blood (occult blood) in the stool specimen. Another blood test for the protein carcinoembryonic antigen (CEA) will be made. This tumor marker is elevated in approximately 28 percent of patients with early colon and rectal cancers.

Special Laboratory Tests   Follow-up diagnostic tests when the history, physical examination, stool tests, and blood tests indicate possible cancer include the use of various "scopes": colonoscopes, proctoscopes, and sigmoidoscopes. These instruments are inserted into the rectum and colon to visualize tumor masses directly. Fortunately, the most common masses seen are polyps, which are premalignant growths but may contain cancer cells from the lining of the bowel. During these procedures, which are performed while the patient is under local or general anesthesia, the physician is able to observe and cut out a small polyp, or to obtain a biopsy of a tumor on the surface of the colon. The biopsy will be examined by a pathologist to determine whether the excised tissue is benign or malignant.

Another useful diagnostic test is the *barium enema*. A solution containing barium is introduced into the colon by means of an enema. A series of X-ray examinations of the patient's abdomen are then taken over a period of an hour. Any masses in the colon will appear as dark shadows in the X-ray film; the barium, which does not allow X rays to penetrate to the film, outlines the colon as a white tube. If cancer is present, and before surgical or other treatment is begun, it is important to conduct a "metastatic workup" as described for lung cancer, including radioactive scans and CT scans to detect spread of the cancer to the liver or other organs.

Although not all of these tests are required for each patient, enough of them must be performed to obtain a specific diagnosis upon which all future therapy will be based.

Stages of Colon Cancer

If colon cancer is diagnosed, the physician will then determine whether the cancer cells have spread to other parts of the body in order to plan specific treatment. The stages of colon cancer are named as follows:

STAGE 0	Carcinoma *in situ*. Very early cancer, found only in the top lining of the colon.
STAGE I	Cancer has spread beyond the top lining of the colon to the second and third layers and involves the inside wall of the colon but has not spread to the outer wall of the colon or outside the colon. Stage I colon cancer is sometimes called Dukes A colon cancer (after the staging system described by Dr. C. E. Dukes in 1932).
STAGE II	Cancer has spread outside the colon to nearby tissues, but has not spread into the lymph nodes. Stage II colon cancer is sometimes called Dukes B colon cancer.
STAGE III	Cancer has spread to nearby lymph nodes but has not spread to other parts of the body. Stage III colon cancer is sometimes called Dukes C colon cancer.
STAGE IV	Cancer has spread to other parts of the body. Stage IV colon cancer is sometimes called Dukes D colon cancer.
RECURRENT	Cancer has come back after it has been treated. It may come back in the colon or in another part of the body. Recurrent cancer of the colon is often found in the liver and/ or lungs.

Treatment of Colon and Rectal Cancers

Both colon and rectal cancers can often be treated successfully and cured with current therapy. Such success stories, of course, are for the cancers that are detected in early stages, before they have spread. Treatment varies with the stage of the disease encountered. Surgery is the most common treatment for all stages of colon cancer. The physician may take out the cancer from the colon using one of the following techniques:

If the cancer is found at a very early stage, the surgeon may take it out without cutting into the abdomen but by putting a tube through the rectum into the colon and cutting the tumor out. This is called *local excision*. If the cancer is found in a small bulging piece of tissue (called a polyp), the operation is called a *polypectomy*.

If the cancer is larger, the surgeon will take out the cancer and a small amount of healthy tissue around it. The healthy parts of the colon are then sewn together (anastomosed). If only a small amount of tissue is removed this is called a *wedge resection*. If a larger amount of tissue is removed, this is called a *bowel resection*.

The surgeon will also take out lymph nodes near the intestine and look at them under the microscope to see whether they contain the cancer. If the surgeon is not able to sew the colon back together, he or she will make an opening (stoma) on the outside of the body for waste to pass out of the body. This is called a *colostomy*. Sometimes the colostomy is needed only until the colon has healed, and then it can be reversed. In other cases, the surgeon may have to take out the entire lower colon, and the colostomy is permanent. Any patient with a colostomy will need to wear a special bag to collect body wastes. This special bag, which sticks to the skin around the stoma with a special glue, can be thrown away after it is used. This bag does not show under clothing, and most people need no special help to maintain it.

Radiation therapy, chemotherapy, or biological therapy may be given in addition to surgery for colon cancer.

Any treatment for cancer of the colon depends on the stage of the disease and the patient's age and general health. The patient may receive a treatment that is considered standard based on its effectiveness in a number of patients in past studies, or may choose to go into a clinical trial. Not all patients are cured with standard therapy, and some standard treatments have undesirable side effects. Clinical trials are designed to find better ways to treat cancer patients and are based on the most up-to-date information. Clinical trials are taking place in most parts of the country for most stages of cancer of the colon. For more information, call the Cancer Information Service at 1-800-4-CANCER.

TREATMENT BY STAGE

STAGE 0

Treatment may be one of the following:
1. Local excision or simple polypectomy.
2. Wedge resection.

STAGE I

Treatment is usually surgery (bowel resection) to remove the cancer.

STAGE II

Treatment is usually surgery (bowel resection) to remove the cancer. If the tumor has spread to nearby tissue, the patient may also receive chemotherapy or radiotherapy following surgery. Clinical trials are evaluating new combinations of chemotherapy drugs or biological agents. Clinical trials are also evaluating radiation therapy following surgery.

STAGE III

Treatment is usually surgery (bowel resection) to remove the cancer followed by chemotherapy. Clinical trials are evaluating new combinations of chemotherapy drugs or biological agents. Clinical trials are also evaluating radiation therapy following surgery with or without chemotherapy or biological therapy.

STAGE IV

Treatment may be one of the following:
1. Surgery (bowel resection) to remove the cancer or to make the colon go around the cancer so that it can still function.
2. Surgery to remove parts of other organs such as the liver, lungs, or ovaries, where the cancer may have spread.
3. Radiation therapy to relieve symptoms.
4. Chemotherapy.

5. Clinical trials of chemotherapy or biological therapy.

RECURRENT   If the cancer has come back in only one
part of the body, treatment may consist of
an operation to take out the cancer. If the
cancer has spread to several parts of the
body, the physician may give either chemotherapy or radiation therapy. The patient
may choose to participate in a clinical trial
testing new chemotherapy drugs or biological therapy.

To learn more about colon cancer, call the National Cancer Institute's Cancer Information Service at 1-800-4-CANCER. The Cancer
Information Service can also send the following free booklets about
cancer of the colon:

What You Need to Know About Cancer of the Colon and Rectum
Research Report: Colon and Rectum

Much of what has been described for cancer of the colon also applies
to cancer of the rectum, which is also part of the body's digestive
system. The last 8 to 10 inches of the colon is called the rectum. The
screening and diagnosis of cancer of the rectum are the same as for
cancer of the colon, but the stages are different.

Stages of Rectal Cancer

STAGE C   Carcinoma *in situ*. Very early cancer, found
only in the top lining of the rectum.

STAGE 1   Cancer has spread beyond the top lining of
the rectum to the second and third layers
and involves the inside wall of the rectum,
but has not spread to the outer wall of the
rectum or outside the rectum. Stage I cancer of the rectum is sometimes called
Dukes A rectal cancer.

STAGE II   Cancer has spread outside the rectum to
nearby tissue, but has not gone into the

	lymph nodes. Stage II cancer of the rectum is sometimes called Dukes B rectal cancer.
STAGE III	Cancer has spread to nearby lymph nodes, but has not spread to other parts of the body. Stage III cancer of the rectum is sometimes called Dukes C rectal cancer.
STAGE IV	Cancer has spread to other parts of the body. Stage IV cancer of the rectum is sometimes called Dukes D rectal cancer.
RECURRENT	Cancer has come back after it has been treated. It may come back in the rectum or in another part of the body. Recurrent cancer of the rectum is often found in the liver and/or lungs.

Treatment of Rectal Cancer

Surgery is the most common treatment for all stages of cancer of the rectum and is the same as that for colon cancer, with the addition of high-energy electricity, called *electrofulguration.* Radiation therapy, chemotherapy, and biological therapy may be given in addition to surgical therapy for rectal cancer.

TREATMENT BY STAGE

STAGE 0	Treatment may be one of the following:
	1. Local excision.
	2. Wedge resection.
	3. Clinical trials of local excision and radiation therapy.
	4. Clinical trials of electrofulguration.
	5. Clinical trials of internal radiation therapy.
STAGE I	Treatment is usually surgery (bowel resection) to remove the cancer. Other treatments that may be chosen, depending on the size and location of the cancer, include:
	1. Internal radiation therapy.
	2. Electrofulguration.

3. Local resection.
4. Clinical trials of radiation and chemotherapy.

STAGE II

Treatment may be one of the following:

1. Surgery (bowel resection) to remove the cancer, followed by radiation therapy and chemotherapy.
2. Surgery (bowel resection) to remove the cancer as well as the colon, rectum, prostate, or bladder, depending on where the cancer has spread. Surgery is followed by radiation and chemotherapy.
3. Radiation therapy followed by surgery (bowel resection) followed by chemotherapy.
4. Clinical trials are evaluating all these treatments to find better combinations of chemotherapy drugs and better ways of combining radiation therapy with chemotherapy.
5. Clinical trials of radiation therapy given during surgery.
6. Clinical trials of biological therapy given following surgery.

STAGE III

Treatment may be one of the following:

1. Surgery (bowel resection) to remove the cancer, followed by radiation therapy and chemotherapy.
2. Surgery (bowel resection) to remove the cancer, as well as the colon, rectum, prostate, or bladder, depending on where the cancer has spread. Surgery is followed by radiation and chemotherapy.
3. Radiation therapy followed by surgery (bowel resection) followed by chemotherapy.
4. Clinical trials are evaluating all these treatments to find better combinations of chemotherapy drugs and better ways

| | of combining radiation therapy with chemotherapy. |

5. Clinical trials of radiation therapy given during surgery.

STAGE IV   Treatment may be one of the following:

1. Surgery (bowel resection) to remove the cancer.
2. If the cancer has spread only to the liver, lungs, or ovaries, surgery to take out the cancer where it has spread.
3. Radiation therapy.
4. Chemotherapy (clinical trials are testing new chemotherapy drugs).

RECURRENT   If the cancer has recurred in only one part of the body, treatment may be an operation to take out the cancer. If the cancer has spread to several parts of the body, the physician may give either chemotherapy or radiation therapy. The patient may also choose to participate in a clinical trial testing new chemotherapy drugs or biological therapy.

To learn more about rectal cancer, call the National Cancer Institute's Cancer Information Service at 1-800-4-CANCER. The Cancer Information Service can also send the following free booklets about rectal cancer:

What You Need to Know About Cancer of the Colon and Rectum
Research Report: Colon and Rectum

The following chart summarizes the current facts about colon and rectal cancers.

COLON AND RECTAL CANCERS

STATUS	155,000 new cases in 1990
	Runs in families at least 10% of the time
	Second most common cancer
	Comprises approximately 15% of all cancers diagnosed
INCIDENCE	Increased approximately 10% between 1973 and 1987
MORTALITY	Decreased approximately 1.5% between 1973 and 1987
KNOWN CAUSES	Animal fat in diet
	Low fiber in diet
POSSIBLE CAUSES	Alcohol, sedentary lifestyle
LIFESTYLE CHANGES TO PREVENT THE CANCER	Reduce consumption of animal fat
	Increase consumption of fiber
	Reduce consumption of alcohol
	Increase exercise
MEDICAL INTERVENTION	Encourage lifestyle changes above
	Regular physical examinations of older men and women and testing stool specimens for presence of blood
	Eventually routine assays for alterations in oncogenes *(ras)* and tumor-suppressor genes (p53, DCC, and APC)
RESEARCH FRONTIERS	Chemoprevention studies are ongoing in patients with colon cancer, polyps, or adenomas of the colon. These studies are using beta-carotene, aspirin, peroxican, ascorbic acid, alpha-tocopherol, and sulindac.
	Individuals with a strong family history of colon or rectal cancer should have sigmoidoscopy annually and tests for blood in bowel movements twice annually.
	Individuals at risk for an inherited form of cancer (Lynch Syndrome)

should have a colonoscopy annually, beginning at age 25.

Patients with familial adenomatous polyposis (about 1% of colon and rectal cancers) should have an annual sigmoidoscopy beginning at age 10; most develop polyps during their teens and have their colons removed surgically by age 20.

Various clinical trials with new chemotherapeutic and biological agents are ongoing. The results of one trial indicate that in high-risk rectal cancer, after surgical excision of the cancer a combination of radiation therapy and 5-fluouracil increases survival and decreases recurrence of the cancer.

Studies are under way to determine if experimental introduction of p53, APC, or DCC genes into human colon cancer cells would convert them to normal cells.

Studies are evaluating the role of tumor-suppressor gene HNPCC in the inherited form of colon cancer (hereditary nonpolyposis colon cancer).

Chapter 11

Breast Cancer

Breast cancer is the third most common cancer in the United States, striking one of every nine American women and causing the deaths of about one-third of its victims. It is most commonly detected by women themselves, as a visible or palpable lump or thickening in the breast tissue. Although quite uncommon, breast cancer does occur in men as well, usually first detected by feeling or seeing a lump in the breast. Breast cancer may also cause retraction of the nipple or discharge, especially bloody discharge, from the nipple. Skin changes such as dimpling, resembling the skin of an orange, as well as redness, tenderness, pain, and increased heat of the skin and underlying tissue are also signs of breast cancer.

Each breast has fifteen to twenty sections called *lobes*, which have many smaller sections called *lobules*. The lobes and lobules are connected by thin tubes called *ducts*. The most common type of breast cancer is *ductal cancer*. It is found in the cells of the ducts. Cancer that begins in the lobes or lobules is called *lobular carcinoma*. Lobular carcinoma is more often found in both breasts than are other types of breast cancer. Inflammatory breast cancer is another, uncommon type of breast cancer. In this disease, the breast is warm, red, and swollen. Like most cancers, breast cancer is best treated when found early.

Screening

Women should feel their breasts each month to search for any lumps or thick areas. They should immediately see their doctor if they notice any changes in their breasts detected by this self-examination.

Screening for breast cancer by special X rays called *mammograms* is now recommended for women forty years of age and older, to be repeated every two to three years. Such screening offers a marvelous improvement in diagnosis, often leading to 85 percent successful early treatment of small tumors (Henderson et al. 1991, p. 1,132). This has resulted in a reduction in breast cancer deaths of about 25 percent (Harris et al. 1992).

Should women between forty and fifty have annual mammograms? Some unconfirmed studies suggest that such regular mammograms actually increase breast cancer mortality in this age group. The value of mammograms in women over fifty years of age has not been questioned, and some experts feel it would be tragic if younger women were dissuaded from having mammograms because of the mistaken results from a flawed study (Allison 1992, p. 1,128).

B. Healy has also argued persuasively against the proposal in the Clinton Health Security Act to discontinue funding for screening mammographies for women in their forties "as if by imperial edict." This governmental dictate is contrary to the recommendations of the American Cancer Society, the American Medical Association, and breast cancer advocacy groups.

The following list explains screening, diagnosis, and examination.

Diagnosis

Symptoms

Most common symptom is a lump or thickening of breast

Discharge from the nipple

Retraction of the nipple

Change in skin of breast, such as dimpling or puckering (like an orange peel)

Redness, swelling, feeling of heat

Physical Examination

Lump in breast

Other physical signs listed above

Enlarged lymph nodes under the arm indicating metastases

Routine Laboratory Tests

Blood tests for general health status, anemia, infections, blood-clotting capacity

Liver function tests to determine whether cancer has spread to liver (Although the cancer can spread to other organs, the liver can be tested for loss of function due to metastasis.)

Electrocardiogram to evaluate heart function

Chest X ray to visualize cancer and enlarged lymph nodes

Special Laboratory Tests   To diagnose the specific type of cancer and to "stage" it—that is, to determine whether it has spread to other organs such as the liver, bone, lungs, or brain.

MAMMOGRAPHY   This soft tissue X ray must be done to help confirm the diagnosis and the extent of the cancer.

ASPIRATION OR SURGICAL BIOPSY   If there is a lump in the breast, the physician may need to cut out a small piece and examine it under the microscope to look for cancer cells. This *biopsy* is sometimes done by inserting a needle into the breast and drawing out *(aspirating)* some fluid and a small amount of tissue; it may also be done by a simple surgical operation to remove a small sample of the tissue in the lump or, if the lump is small, the entire mass.

Depending on the pathologist's report of the biopsied tissue— and it must be emphasized that 80 percent of lumps in breast tissue are not cancerous, but rather cystic or fibrous lumps—additional diagnostic tests are in order.

ESTROGEN AND PROGESTERONE RECEPTOR TESTS   If the biopsy shows cancer, it is important that estrogen and progesterone receptor tests be done on the cancer cells. These tests can tell whether hormones affect how the cancer grows. They can also give information about the chances of the tumor recurring. The results help the physician decide whether to use hormone therapy to stop the cancer from growing. (Tissue from the tumor needs to be taken to the laboratory for estrogen and progesterone receptor tests at the time of biopsy because it may be hard to get enough cancer cells later.)

METASTATIC WORKUP   If the biopsied tissue is cancerous, before any treatment is planned it is imperative to conduct a series of tests to determine whether the cancer has spread to other sites in the body. This metastatic workup consists of radioactive scans of bone, liver, and other organs. In these painless scans, various radionu-clides, including gallium, are injected into a vein and then looked for throughout the body by scanning for radioactive emissions. The radioactive substances are "taken up" by rapidly dividing cells in tumor tissue more readily than in the cells of normal tissues. They are sensitive indicators of bone metastases. Also useful in some patients is an ultrasound scan, which can sometimes localize metastatic cancer tissue; it reflects the sound waves differently than do normal tissues.

Although not all of these tests are required for each patient, enough of them must be performed to obtain a specific diagnosis upon which all future therapy will be based.

A patient's chance of recovery and course of treatment depend on the stage of the cancer (the size of the tumor and whether it is just in the breast or has spread to other places in the body), the type of cancer, certain characteristics of the cancer cells, and the patient's age, menopausal status, and general state of health.

The prognosis of breast cancers that have not spread to lymph nodes is also related to the size of the tumor: about a 10 percent risk of relapse for each 1 centimeter of tumor. Thus a patient with a 2.5-centimeter tumor (1 inch in diameter) has about a 25 percent chance of relapse. When the cancer has spread to lymph nodes, the chance of recurrence is higher.

Stages of Breast Cancer

Once breast cancer has been diagnosed, more tests will be done to find out whether it has spread to other parts of the body. This is called *staging*. The physician needs to know the stage of the patient's disease in order to plan treatment. The stages of breast cancer are named as follows:

IN SITU	About 5 to 10 percent of breast cancers are discovered very early. They are sometimes called carcinoma *in situ* (found only in the local area, without going to nearby tissues). Other terms for this type of breast cancer are intraductal carcinoma or ductal carcinoma *in situ* and lobular carcinoma *in situ*.
STAGE I	Cancer is no bigger than 2 centimeters (just under 1 inch) and has not spread beyond the breast.
STAGE II	Any of the following may be true of stage II breast cancer:
	Cancer is no bigger than 2 centimeters but

has spread to the lymph nodes under the arm (the axillary lymph nodes).

Cancer is between 2 and 5 centimeters (from 1 to 2 inches) and may or may not have spread to the lymph nodes under the arm.

Cancer is bigger than 5 centimeters (larger than 2 inches) but has not spread to the lymph nodes under the arm.

STAGE III
Stage IIIA is defined by either of the following:

Cancer is smaller than 5 centimeters and has spread to the lymph nodes under the arm, which have grown into each other or into other structures and are attached to them.

Cancer is bigger than 5 centimeters and has spread to the lymph nodes under the arm.

Stage IIIB is defined by either of the following:

Cancer has spread to tissues near the breast (chest wall, including the ribs and the muscles in the chest).

Cancer has spread to lymph nodes near the collarbone.

STAGE IV
Cancer has spread to other organs of the body.

INFLAMMATORY
This special class of breast cancer is rare. The breast looks as if it is inflamed because of its red appearance and warmth. The skin may show signs of ridges and wheals or it may have a pitted appearance. Inflammatory breast cancer tends to spread quickly.

RECURRENT
Cancer has come back after it has been treated. It may come back in the breast, in the muscles of the chest (the chest wall), or in another part of the body.

Treatment of Breast Cancer

Many articles appear in the lay press about the results of clinical trials of different treatments for breast cancer. The excellent method for detection by mammography of small lesions, well before they have spread or even sometimes before they are palpable, has allowed the use of much more limited surgery to remove the cancer in some instances—removal of just the lump, or *lumpectomy*, and the more conservative use of radiation therapy with or without chemotherapy or hormone therapy. This encouraging situation is not always the case, however, and some women still do not seek medical aid for breast cancer until it is a large tumor and has spread to local lymph nodes and distant sites.

Four types of treatment are available for all patients with breast cancer: surgery, radiation therapy, chemotherapy, and hormone therapy (using hormones to stop the cells from growing). Biological therapy (using your body's immune system to fight cancer) and bone marrow transplantation are being tested in clinical trials.

Surgery has a role in the treatment of most patients with breast cancer. It is used to take out the cancer from the breast. Usually, some of the lymph nodes under the arm are also taken out and examined under the microscope for cancer cells. Any of a number of different procedures may be used for treatment:

Lumpectomy (sometimes called excisional biopsy) takes out only the lump itself. It is usually followed by radiation therapy to the rest of the breast. Most physicians also take out some of the lymph nodes under the arm.

Partial or *segmental mastectomy* takes out the cancer, some of the breast tissue around it, and the lining over the chest muscle. Usually some of the lymph nodes under the arm are also taken out. In most cases radiation therapy follows.

Total or *simple mastectomy* removes the whole breast. Sometimes lymph nodes under the arm are also taken out.

Modified radical mastectomy takes out the breast, some of the lymph nodes under the arm, and the lining over the chest muscles (but leaves the muscles). This is the most common operation for breast cancer.

Radical mastectomy (also called the Halsted radical mastectomy) takes out the breast, the chest muscles, and all of the lymph nodes under the arm. This was the main operation for many years, but is used now only when the tumor has spread to the chest muscles.

If a woman is going to have a mastectomy, she may want to think about having breast reconstruction (making a new breast). It may be done at the time of the mastectomy or at some future time. The breast may be made with the patient's own tissue or by using implants. Different types of implants can be used. Recently, the Food and Drug Administration (FDA) requested that breast implants filled with silicone gel not be used until the FDA can determine their safety. Saline-filled breast implants, which contain salt water rather than silicone gel, may be used, however.

Radiation therapy uses high-energy X rays to kill cancer cells and shrink tumors. Radiation may come from a machine outside the body (external radiation therapy) or from putting materials that produce radiation (radiosotopes) through thick plastic tubes in the area where the cancer cells are found (internal radiation therapy).

Chemotherapy uses drugs to kill cancer cells. Chemotherapy may be taken by mouth or it may be put into the body by a needle in a vein or a muscle. Chemotherapy is called a systemic treatment because the drugs enter the bloodstream, travel through the body, and can kill cancer cells outside the breast area.

Hormone therapy is used to stop the hormones in the body that help cancer grow. This may be done by using drugs that change the way hormones work or by surgery that takes out organs that make hormones, such as the ovaries. Like chemotherapy, hormone therapy can act on cells all over the body.

If the doctor removes all the cancer that can be seen at the time of the operation, radiation therapy, chemotherapy, or hormone therapy may be given after surgery to kill any cancer cells that are left. Therapy given after an operation when there are no discernible cancer cells is called *adjuvant therapy*.

Biological therapy (sometimes called biological response modifier [BRM] therapy or immunotherapy) tries to get the patient's own body to fight the cancer. Materials made by the patient's body or made in a laboratory may be able to boost, direct, or restore the body's natural defenses against disease.

Bone marrow transplantation is a newer type of treatment. Sometimes breast cancer becomes resistant to treatment with radiation therapy or chemotherapy. Very high doses of chemotherapy may then be used to treat it. But these high doses can destroy a person's marrow, so marrow is taken from various bones and frozen before the treatment begins. The patient is given high-dose chemotherapy with or without radiation therapy. Then the marrow that was removed is thawed and returned to the patient intravenously to replace the marrow that was destroyed. This type of transplant is called an *autologous* transplant.

A breast cancer patient may receive treatment that is considered standard based on its effectiveness in a number of patients in past studies, or she may choose to go into a clinical trial. Not all patients are cured with standard therapy, and some standard treatments may have undesirable side effects. Clinical trials are designed to find better ways to treat cancer patients and are based on the most up-to-date information. Clinical trials are taking place in most parts of the country for all stages of breast cancer. For more information, call the Cancer Information Service at 1-800-4-CANCER.

TREATMENT BY STAGE

In situ

Treatment depends on whether the patient has ductal or lobular cancer. If it is ductal cancer, treatment may be one of the following:

Total mastectomy.

Lumpectomy followed by radiation therapy.

Some of the lymph nodes under the arm may also be removed during these surgeries. Clinical trials are testing surgery to remove the cancer and part of the breast (partial or segmental mastectomy).

If the cancer is lobular carcinoma *in situ*, the patient has a higher risk of getting an invasive cancer in both breasts. Not all physicians agree on how lobular carcinoma *in situ* should be treated. Treatment may be one of the following:

Biopsy to remove the cancer, followed by regular examinations and mammograms to make sure the patient does not develop another cancer.

| | Surgery to remove one or both breasts (total mastectomy). Lymph nodes under the arm may or may not be taken out. |
| STAGE I | Treatment may be one of the following: |

Lumpectomy followed by radiation therapy. Some of the lymph nodes under the arm are also removed.

Partial or segmental mastectomy and removal of some of the lymph nodes under the arm. Radiation therapy is given following surgery.

Total mastectomy or modified radical mastectomy. Some of the lymph nodes under the arm are also taken out.

Chemotherapy or hormone therapy may be given in addition to these treatments. Clinical trials are testing new chemotherapy drugs, combinations of drugs, and new ways of giving chemotherapy.

| STAGE II | Treatment may be one of the following: |

Lumpectomy followed by radiation therapy. Some of the lymph nodes under the arm are also removed.

Partial or segmental mastectomy and removal of some of the lymph nodes under the arm. Radiation therapy is given following surgery.

Total mastectomy or modified radical mastectomy. Some of the lymph nodes under the arm are also taken out.

Radical mastectomy. This operation is used only in special situations.

Following surgery, chemotherapy and/or hormonal therapy may be given. Clinical trials are testing new chemotherapy and hormonal drugs, new drug combinations, and new ways of giving chemotherapy.

Clinical trials are also testing no chemotherapy or hormonal therapy for certain patients. In some cases, adjuvant radiation therapy may be given to the chest following mastectomy to reduce the risk of recurrence.

STAGE III

If the patient has stage IIIA (operable) cancer, treatment may be one of the following:

Modified radical mastectomy. Some of the lymph nodes under the arm are also taken out.

Radical mastectomy.

Radiation therapy is given before or after surgery. Chemotherapy with or without hormone therapy is given following surgery. Clinical trials are testing new chemotherapy and hormonal drugs, new drug combinations, and new ways of giving chemotherapy.

If the patient has stage IIIB cancer (cannot be operated on and includes inflammatory breast cancer), treatment will probably be biopsy followed by radiation therapy to the breast and the lymph nodes. A mastectomy may be done following radiation therapy. Chemotherapy or hormonal therapy may be given before or after surgery and radiation therapy. Clinical trials are testing new chemotherapy drugs and biological therapy, new drug combinations, and new ways of giving chemotherapy.

STAGE IV

Treatment will probably be biopsy followed by radiation therapy or mastectomy. Hormonal therapy or chemotherapy will probably also be given. Clinical trials are testing new chemotherapy and hormonal drugs and new combinations of drugs.

INFLAMMATORY

Treatment will probably be a combination of chemotherapy, hormonal therapy, and radiation therapy, maybe followed by surgery to remove the breast. The treatment is usually similar to that for stage IIIB or IV breast cancer.

RECURRENT

Breast cancer that recurs can often be treated but usually cannot be cured. The patient's choice of treatment depends on hormone receptor levels, the previous kind of treatment, the length of time between first treatment and recurrence, where the cancer recurred, whether the patient still menstruates, and other factors. Treatment may be one of the following:

For the small group of patients whose cancer has come back in only one place, surgery and/or radiation therapy.

Radiation therapy to help relieve pain due to the spread of the cancer to the bones and other places.

Chemotherapy or hormonal therapy.

A clinical trial of new chemotherapy drugs, new hormonal drugs, biological therapy, or bone marrow transplantation.

To learn more about breast cancer, call the National Cancer Institute's Information Service at 1-800-4-CANCER. The Cancer Information Service can also send the following free booklets about breast cancer:

After Breast Cancer: A Guide to Followup Care
Breast Biopsy: What You Should Know
Breast Cancer: Understanding Treatment Options
Breast Reconstruction: A Matter of Choice
Mastectomy: A Treatment for Breast Cancer
Radiation Therapy: A Treatment for Early Stage Breast Cancer
What You Need to Know About Breast Cancer

For information on breast implants, write: Breast Implants, Food and Drug Administration, HFE-88, Rockville, MD 20857. The FDA also has a hotline to answer questions about silicone gel–filled breast implants. Call 1-800-532-4440, Monday through Friday, 9:00 A.M. to 7:00 P.M. (Eastern Standard Time).

The following chart summarizes the current facts about breast cancer.

BREAST CANCER

STATUS	150,900 new cases in the United States during 1990
	Second most common cause of death from cancer in women, after lung cancer
	Up to 30% runs in families
	Accounts for approximately 15% of all cancer diagnosed in 1990
INCIDENCE	Increased approximately 24% between 1973 and 1987
MORTALITY	Increased approximately 2% between 1973 and 1987
KNOWN CAUSE	Ovarian hormones; estrogens and progesterone
POSSIBLE CAUSES	Alcohol, obesity in postmenopausal women
LIFESTYLE CHANGES TO PREVENT THE CANCER	Reduce the use of estrogen and progesterone in postmenopausal women
	Reduce alcohol consumption and obesity
MEDICAL INTERVENTION	Evaluate the necessity of using estrogen-replacement therapy and progesterone in postmenopausal women
	Encourage reduction in obesity and alcohol consumption
	Close attention to family history of breast cancer
	Routine use of mammograms in women over 40
	Eventually test for alterations in oncogenes (erb B, *neu*, HER-2, and *myc*) and tumor-suppressor genes (p53, RB, and those on chromosomes 3 and 11)
	25% to 30% of patients who have overactive oncogenes (erb, *neu*, HER-2) are more likely to relapse than patients with a normally active gene.

RESEARCH FRONTIERS

Taxol, a very promising new anticancer drug, will be tested on breast cancer patients.

NCI will soon launch a 16,000-member clinical trial in the United States and Canada on the drug tamoxifen, an estrogen suppressor, to determine whether women who have had cancer in one breast can have fewer recurrences and avoid it in the other breast.

The p53 tumor-suppressor gene is noted to be defective in patients in family clusters of breast cancer at an early age.

Loss of function of p53 (an increase in p53 mutant protein) is under study as a marker for poor prognosis. Studies are evaluating the presence of antibodies against p53 protein in patients' serum as a diagnostic and prognostic marker.

Studies are under way to isolate BRCAI, a breast cancer susceptibility gene, on chromosome 17; also to evaluate its use as a screening marker in women at high risk for breast cancer.

Only 30% of breast cancer cases are now linked to oncogenes, tumor-suppressor genes, alcohol, and obesity.

The NCI has spent over $1 billion on breast cancer since the National Cancer Act of 1971; excellent progress has been made in improved treatment and research findings, but limited success has been achieved in reducing mortality from the disease.

Chapter 12

Prostate Cancer

PROSTATE CANCER IS THE SCOURGE OF OLDER MEN, ESPECIALLY BLACK men. Death due to prostate cancer is twice as high in black men in the United States than in white men. For unknown reasons, this cancer continues to increase each year at an alarming rate. During the last decade, it has become the most common newly diagnosed cancer in men in the United States. One out of eleven men develop it, mostly after age sixty-five. It begins to increase in incidence after age forty until it becomes the most common cause of cancer death in men over seventy-five years old. It is the third most common cause of cancer death in men, in general (after lung and colon cancer), accounting for 11 percent of deaths, totaling 28,000 per year (Henderson et al. 1991). Prostate cancer is not related to smoking.

At a recent Cancer Symposium, the speaker dramatically stated that one-third of all the men in the audience over fifty had prostate cancer in hidden or latent form. At present it is estimated that ten million males in the United States have this silent form of prostate cancer. It is unknown how or when the latent form is activated to the aggressive form, but it is possible that environmental factors play a role. For instance, Japanese men have about the same prevalence of the latent form as do men in the United States. Only a few of the latent cancers in Japanese men are activated to the aggressive form, however, while such an activation is more common in males in the United States, especially as they age. Curiously, when Japanese males migrate to the United States, their latent cancers are commonly activated to a rate approaching the high levels observed in the United States. Which environmental factors in the United States—dietary, carcinogens, others—might cause this activation remains unknown. New advances permit earlier diagnosis of prostate cancer, and, if it has not spread, curative therapy is available.

In cancer of the prostate, cancer cells are found in the prostate, a male sex gland located just below the bladder and in front of the rectum. About the size of a walnut, the prostate surrounds part of the urethra, the tube that carries urine from the bladder to the outside of the body. The prostate makes fluid that becomes part of the semen, the white fluid that contains sperm.

As men age, their prostates may get bigger and block the urethra or the bladder, which can cause them to have difficulty urinating or may interfere with sexual function. This condition is called benign prostatic hyperplasia (BPH), and, although it is not cancer, it may require surgery to correct it. The symptoms of BPH or of other problems in the prostate may be similar to symptoms of prostate cancer.

Screening

The most important screening technique is an annual rectal examination after age forty. Also newly recommended is an annual blood test for the presence of a "marker" of prostate cancer called prostate specific antigen, or PSA. Studies have indicated that the combination of rectal examination and measurement of the blood PSA is the best method for detecting this cancer. About 12,000 prostate cancers are detected each year while they are still curable.

To do the rectal examination, the physician will insert a gloved finger into the rectum to feel for lumps in the prostate. An ultrasound, which uses sound waves to make a picture of the bladder, may also be done.

Diagnosis

Symptoms The symptoms of prostate cancer are mainly problems of urination caused when the prostate gland, enlarged by cancer, begins to block the urethra, the tube that carries urine through the penis. This blockage, initially partial, causes the bladder to retain urine, thus the frequent feeling of urgency to urinate, especially at night. It may be difficult to start or stop urination, and the stream of urine may be narrow.

The bladder is not emptying completely, and the backed-up urine sometimes becomes infected, causing burning, painful urination of cloudy, sometimes bloody urine. Tenderness over the bladder and a dull ache in the pelvis and back may occur. Undiagnosed but advanced prostate cancer can even cause bone pain because of the spread to bones. Often there are no symptoms of early prostate cancer.

Fortunately, the most common cause of prostatic enlargement and the resultant urinary symptoms just described is benign prostatic hypertrophy, a nonmalignant enlargement of the prostate. Approximately half of men over fifty years of age have such an enlargement of the prostate. It must be remembered, however, that benign prostatic hypertrophy and prostate cancer can both be found in the same patient, and only a thorough diagnostic workup can determine the correct diagnosis. Another disease, an inflammation of the prostate gland called prostatitis, may also have the same symptoms.

Physical Examination   After eliciting a health history suggestive of prostate cancer, the physician will make a complete physical examination that includes a digital rectal examination. Prostate cancer can often be felt as an enlarged prostate gland that is sometimes hard and nodular.

Routine Laboratory Tests   Routine laboratory tests of blood and urine and a chest X ray are obtained. PSA is a powerful new blood test that distinguishes prostate cancer from benign prostatic hypertrophy. This test is now routine and, if high levels of the PSA marker are detected, is very suggestive that cancer of the prostate is present. Another blood test is for an enzyme called prostatic acid phosphatase. This enzyme is made by the prostate and also aids in diagnosis, as do other tests for serum and phosphatase and serum alkaline phosphatase.

Special Laboratory Tests

Examination of urine and prostatic secretions for cancer cells.

Massaging of prostate gland by a finger inserted in the rectum, following which urine and prostatic secretion specimens can be obtained and examined under the microscope for the presence of cancer cells.

Another important new test that helps differentiate between prostate cancer and benign prostatic hypertrophy is called transrectal sonography. In this simple procedure, an ultrasound probe is inserted into the rectum and can detect lesions as small as ¼ inch in diameter.

The transrectal sonography instrument also has a probe that can guide a biopsy needle to the tissue to be extracted. A new biopsy technique with a small needle in a "biopsy gun" can be used to obtain biopsies, under anesthesia, through the rectum or peritoneum.

Magnetic resonance imaging also helps differentiate among prostate cancer, benign prostate hypertrophy, and prostatitis. Small probes give such precise images that they make biopsies unnecessary.

If prostate cancer is suspected, a number of needle biopsies of the prostate gland will usually be taken, and the aspirated fluid and tissue stained and examined microscopically by a pathologist to determine whether cancer cells are present. Depending on the results of all these tests, it may be important to obtain a metastatic bone survey by routine X-ray examination, as well as a bone scan. Although not all of these tests are required for each patient, enough of them must be performed to obtain a specific diagnosis upon which all future therapy will be based.

Stages of Prostate Cancer

Once cancer of the prostate has been diagnosed, more tests will be conducted to find out whether cancer cells have spread from the prostate to surrounding tissues or to other parts of the body. This is called staging. The physician needs to know the stage of the disease in order to plan treatment. The stages of prostate cancer are named as follows:

STAGE A	Prostate cancer at this stage cannot be felt and causes no symptoms. The cancer is only in the prostate and is usually found accidentally when surgery is done for other reasons, such as for benign prostatic hypertrophy (BPH).
STAGE A1	Cancer cells are found in only one area of the prostate.
STAGE A2	Cancer cells are found in many areas of the prostate.
STAGE B	The tumor can be felt in the prostate during a rectal examination, but cancer cells are found only in the prostate gland.
STAGE C	Cancer cells have spread outside the

	covering (capsule) of the prostate to tissues around the prostate. The glands that produce semen (the seminal vesicles) may have cancer in them.
STAGE D	Cancer cells have spread (metastasized) to lymph nodes or to organs and tissues far away from the prostate.
STAGE D1	Cancer cells have spread to lymph nodes near the prostate.
STAGE D2	Cancer cells have spread to lymph nodes far from the prostate or to other parts of the body, such as the bone, liver, or lungs.
RECURRENT	Cancer has come back after it has been treated. It may come back in the prostate or in another part of the body.

Treatment of Prostate Cancer

Cancer of the prostate can usually be cured when it is detected early. But even when it is unsuccessfully treated and merely controlled, many older men die of other causes before the cancer causes discomfort or fatality. Optimum treatment of prostate cancer depends on a number of factors, such as the patient's age and health and the stages of the disease. The three most common forms of therapy are surgical removal of the prostate, radiation therapy, and hormone therapy. The use of chemotherapy and biological therapy (using the body's immune system to fight cancer) in prostate cancer is being studied in clinical trials.

Surgery is a common treatment. The physician may take out the cancer using one of the following operations:

Radical prostatectomy removes the prostate and some of the tissue around it. The surgeon may cut into the space between the scrotum and the anus (the perineum) in an operation called a *perineal prostatectomy*, or may cut into the lower abdomen, called a *retropubic prostatectomy*. Radical prostatectomy is done only if the cancer has not spread outside the prostate. Often the physician will first surgically remove lymph nodes in the pelvis to see whether they contain cancer. This is called a *pelvic lymph node dissection*.

If the lymph nodes contain cancer, usually the surgeon will not do a prostatectomy and may or may not recommend other therapy at this time. Impotence can occur in men who have surgery for prostate cancer.

Transurethral resection cuts cancer from the prostate using a tool with a small wire loop on the end that is put into the prostate through the urethra. This operation is sometimes done to relieve symptoms caused by the tumor before other treatment, or in men who cannot have a radical prostatectomy because of age or other illness.

Radiation therapy uses high-energy X rays to kill cancer cells and shrink tumors. Radiation may come from a machine outside the body (external radiation therapy) or from putting materials that produce radiation (radioisotopes) through thin plastic tubes in the area where the cancer cells are found (internal radiation therapy). Impotence may occur in men treated with radiation therapy.

Hormone therapy uses hormones to stop cancer cells from growing. Hormone therapy for prostate cancer can take several forms. Male hormones (especially testosterone) can help prostate cancer grow. To stop the cancer, female hormones or drugs that decrease the amount of male hormones may be given. Sometimes an operation to remove the testicles (orchiectomy) is performed to stop the testicles from making testosterone. This treatment is usually given to men with advanced prostate cancer. Growth of breast tissue is a common side effect of therapy with female hormones (estrogens); hot flashes can occur after orchiectomy and other hormone therapies.

Chemotherapy uses drugs to kill cancer cells. Chemotherapy may be taken by pill, or it may be put into the body by a needle in a vein or muscle. Chemotherapy is called a systemic treatment because the drug enters the bloodstream, travels through the body, and can kill any cancer cells beyond the area where they have been identified. To date, chemotherapy has not had significant value in treating prostate cancer, but clinical trials are in progress to find more effective drugs.

Biological therapy tries to get the patient's body to fight the cancer. It uses materials made by the body or made in a laboratory to boost, direct, or restore the body's natural defenses against disease. Biological therapy is sometimes called biological response modifier (BRM) therapy or immunotherapy.

Any treatment of prostate cancer depends on the stage of the disease and the patient's age and overall condition. If he does not have any symptoms, the physician may follow him closely without any treatment if he is older or has another, more serious illness.

The patient may receive treatment that is considered standard based on its effectiveness in a number of patients in past clinical trials, or he may choose to go into a clinical trial. Not all patients are cured with standard therapy, and some standard treatments have undesirable side effects. Clinical trials are designed to find better ways to treat cancer patients and are based on the most up-to-date information. Clinical trials are taking place in most parts of the country for most stages of prostate cancer. For more information, call the Cancer Information Service at 1-800-4-CANCER.

TREATMENT BY STAGE

STAGE A1	If the man is older, the physician may follow him closely without any treatment. The physician may choose this option because in this stage the cancer is not causing any symptoms or other problems and may be growing slowly. If the patient is younger, he may undergo surgery to remove the prostate and the tissue around it (radical prostatectomy) or external radiation therapy.
STAGE A2	Treatment may be one of the following:
	1. External radiation therapy.
	2. Surgery to remove the prostate and the tissue around it (radical prostatectomy). Usually some of the lymph nodes in the pelvis are also removed (pelvic lymph node dissection). Radiation therapy may be given after surgery in some cases.
	3. A clinical trial of internal radiation therapy, often in addition to pelvic lymph node dissection.
	4. If the patient is older or has another, more serious illness, the patient may be followed closely without treatment.
STAGE B	Treatment may be one of the following:

1. Radical prostatectomy and usually pelvic lymph node dissection. Radiation therapy may be given following surgery.
2. External radiation therapy. Clinical trials are testing new types of radiation.
3. A clinical trial of internal radiation therapy, often in addition to pelvic lymph node dissection.
4. If the patient is older or has another, more serious illness, the physician may follow him closely without treatment. The physician may choose this option if the cancer is not causing any symptoms or other problems and may be growing slowly.

STAGE C   Treatment may be one of the following:

1. External radiation therapy. Clinical trials are testing new types of radiation.
2. Radical prostatectomy and usually pelvic lymph node dissection. Radiation therapy may be given following surgery.
3. If the patient is older or has another, more serious illness, the physician may follow him closely without treatment. The physician may choose this option if the cancer is not causing any symptoms or other problems and may be growing slowly.
4. A clinical trial of internal radiation therapy, often in addition to pelvic lymph node dissection.

If the patient is unable to have surgery or radiation therapy, the physician may give treatments to relieve symptoms, such as problems urinating. In this case, treatment may be one of the following:

1. Radiation therapy to relieve symptoms.
2. Surgery to cut the cancer from the prostate using a tool with a small wire loop on the end that is put into the prostate

through the urethra (transurethral resection).

3. Hormone therapy.

STAGE D1

Treatment may be one of the following:

1. External-beam radiation therapy. Clinical trials are testing new forms of radiation. Hormone therapy may be given in addition to radiation.

2. Radical prostatectomy and surgery to remove the testicles (orchiectomy).

3. If the patient is older or has another, more serious illness, the physician may follow him closely without treatment. The physician may choose this option because the cancer is not causing any symptoms or other problems and may be growing slowly.

4. A clinical trial of hormone therapy.

STAGE D2

Treatment may be one of the following:

1. Hormone therapy.

2. External-beam radiation therapy to relieve symptoms.

3. Transurethral resection to relieve symptoms.

4. A clinical trial of chemotherapy or new forms of hormone therapy.

5. The physician may follow the patient and wait until he develops symptoms before giving treatment.

RECURRENT

Treatment depends on many things, including what treatment the patient has already had. If he has had surgery to remove the prostate (prostatectomy) and the cancer recurs in only a small area, he may receive radiation therapy. If the disease has spread to other parts of the body, he will probably receive hormone therapy. Radiation therapy may be given to relieve symptoms such as bone pain. The patient may also choose to take part in a clinical trial of chemotherapy or biological therapy.

To learn more about cancer of the prostate, call the National Cancer Institute's Cancer Information Service at 1-800-4-CANCER. The Cancer Information Service can also send the following free booklets about prostate cancer:

What You Need to Know About Prostate Cancer
Research Report: Cancer of the Prostate

The following chart summarizes the current facts about prostate cancer.

PROSTATE CANCER

STATUS
: 106,000 new cases in the United States during 1990
Comprised approximately 10% of all cancers diagnosed in 1990

INCIDENCE
: Increased approximately 45% between 1973 and 1987

MORTALITY
: Increased approximately 7% between 1973 and 1987, proportionately lower than the increased incidence

KNOWN CAUSE
: The male hormone testosterone

POSSIBLE CAUSE
: The female hormone estrogen

LIFESTYLE CHANGES TO PREVENT THE CANCER
: Unfortunately, there are no lifestyle changes that are known to help reduce the risk of prostate cancer.

MEDICAL INTERVENTION
: Educate black men of their high risk for this cancer
Encourage routine rectal examinations in all men over 50 years of age
Encourage testing for prostate specific antigen (PSA) in all men over 50 years of age
Ultrasound examination as required
Eventually assays for alteration in tumor-suppressor genes (Rb and others)

RESEARCH FRONTIERS
: Recently reported studies indicate that radical prostatectomies using the anatomic approach greatly lower the cancer recurrence rate, preserve urinary control in virtually all patients, and preserve sexual function in 68% of all patients (90% of those under 50 years of age) who were sexually potent before the operation.
Prostate-specific antigen is considered to be the first organ-specific serum marker in all of cancer biology. It is an invaluable tool for the clinician.

Chapter 13

Bladder Cancer

IN 1895, BLADDER CANCER WAS NOTED TO OCCUR FOLLOWING EXPOSURE to the aniline dye betanaphthylamine. Since then, it has been associated with exposure to certain other chemicals and the products of tobacco tar that are present in the urine following smoking. Although the incidence of bladder cancer increased approximately 12 percent in the United States from 1973 to 1987, the mortality from the disease decreased by approximately 23 percent. During 1990, 49,000 new cases were diagnosed. Most patients were between fifty and seventy years of age. Men are three times as likely as women to develop it. Bladder cancer accounts for approximately 5 percent of all malignant tumors. Most bladder cancers grow slowly and do not spread to other parts of the body. Although many bladder tumors are found to be benign, they may become malignant.

Several types of bladder cancer are recognized: *papillary* and *transition-cell* cancers are the most common and most easily cured. *Squamous-cell*, less common and more invasive, has a poorer prognosis. *Adenocarcinoma* is rare.

Screening

Routine urinalysis that detects even small amounts of blood in the urine may suggest bladder cancer. Examination of urine for cancer cells in high-risk occupational groups and in areas of schistosomiases (a worm infection) must be evaluated as a secondary tool.

Diagnosis

Symptoms   Blood in the urine, making it look bright red or rusty-colored, is a common first symptom. Other symptoms are pain or burning upon urination, frequent urination, and feeling the need to urinate but nothing comes out. The urine may appear cloudy because it contains pus.

Physical Examination   After taking a health history, the physician will make a physical examination that includes an internal examination by inserting gloved fingers into the rectum and/or vagina to feel for lumps. The physician will also feel for a mass above the pubis.

Routine Laboratory Tests

   Blood tests, urine analyses

   Chest X ray

   Electrocardiogram

Special Laboratory Tests

   Examination of urine for cancer cells.

   Intravenous pyelogram may reveal a tumor or tumors in the bladder. For this test, a special dye containing iodine is given intravenously. The dye goes into the urine, making the bladder easier to see on X rays. Tumors appear as filling defects in the bladder.

   Cystoscopy: An instrument called a cystoscope is inserted into the bladder through the urethra. If tissue that is not normal is seen, the physician will cut out a small piece that can be looked at under the microscope (biopsy) to see whether it contains any cancer cells. Computer tomography (CT) scans of the pelvis, ultrasound, or magnetic resonance imaging (MRI) may be of value in determining the extent of the cancer and whether it has spread to the lymph nodes, lungs, or liver.

   Although not all of these tests are required for each patient, enough of them must be performed to obtain a specific diagnosis upon which all future therapy will be based.

Stages of Bladder Cancer

The physician needs to know the stage of the disease in order to plan appropriate treatment. The stages of bladder cancer are named as follows:

STAGE 0	Carcinoma *in situ*. Very early cancer found only on the inner lining of the bladder. After the cancer is taken out, no swelling or lumps are felt during an internal examination.
STAGE I	Cancer cells have spread a little deeper into the inner lining of the bladder but have not spread to the muscular wall of the bladder.
STAGE II	Cancer cells have spread to the inside lining of the muscles lining the bladder.
STAGE III	Cancer cells have spread throughout the muscular wall of the bladder and/or to the layer of tissue surrounding the bladder. The physician may feel swelling or lumps after surgically removing the cancer.
STAGE IV	Cancer cells have spread to the nearby reproductive organs or to the lymph nodes in the area. The cancer may have also spread to lymph nodes and other places far away from the bladder.
RECURRENT	Cancer has come back after it has been treated. It may come back in the original place or in another part of the body.

Treatment of Bladder Cancer

There are many types and stages of bladder cancer, and treatments vary widely for individual patients. A single papillary tumor can be treated successfully by an electrocautery fulguration to destroy the tissue. A highly malignant and extensive cancer requires extensive surgery, including removal of the bladder. Four kinds of treatment are used: surgery, chemotherapy, radiation therapy, and biological therapy. In addition, a new type of treatment called *photodynamic therapy* is being tested in clinical trials.

In surgery, the urologist may take out the cancer using one of the following operations:

> *Transurethral resection* is an operation that uses a cystoscope inserted into the bladder through the urethra. The urologist then uses a tool with a small wire loop on the end to remove the cancer or to burn the tumor away with high-energy electricity (fulguration).
>
> *Segmental cystectomy* is an operation to take out the part of the bladder where the cancer is found. Because bladder cancer often occurs in more than one part of the bladder, this operation is used only in selected cases where the cancer is in one area.
>
> *Cystectomy* is an operation to take out the bladder.
>
> *Radical cystectomy* is an operation to take out the bladder and the tissue around it. In women, the uterus, ovaries, fallopian tubes, part of the vagina, and urethra are also removed. In men, the prostate and the glands that produce fluid that is part of the semen (seminal vesicles) are also removed, and the urethra may be removed as well. The lymph nodes in the pelvis may also be taken out (pelvic lymph node dissection).
>
> *Urinary diversion* is an operation to make a way for urine to pass out of the body so that it does not go through the bladder. It is used to relieve bladder symptoms when the tumor has spread.

If the bladder is removed, the urologist will need to make a new way for the patient to store and pass urine. There are several ways to do this. Sometimes the urologist will use part of the small intestine to make a tube through which urine can pass out of the body through an opening (stoma) on the outside of the body. This is sometimes called an *ostomy* or *urostomy*. This requires that the patient wear a special bag to collect urine. This special bag, which sticks to the skin around the stoma with a special glue, can be thrown away after it is used. This bag does not show under clothing, and most people need no special help to maintain it. The urologist may also use part of the small intestine to make a new storage pouch (a continent reservoir) inside the body where the urine can collect. With this procedure, a tube (catheter) is needed to drain the urine through the stoma. Newer methods use a part of the small intestine to make a new storage pouch that is connected to the remaining part of the urethra, if it has not been removed. Urine then passes out of the body through the urethra, eliminating the need for a stoma.

Chemotherapy uses drugs to kill cancer cells. Chemotherapy may be taken by pill, or it may be put into the body through a needle in a vein or muscle. Chemotherapy is called a systemic treatment because the drug enters the bloodstream, travels through the body, and can kill cancer cells outside the bladder. Chemotherapy may be given in a fluid that is put into the bladder through a tube going through the urethra (intravesical chemotherapy).

If the urologist removes all the cancer that can be seen at the time of the operation, the patient may be given chemotherapy after surgery to kill any cancer cells that are left. Chemotherapy given after an operation to a person who has no cancer cells that can be seen is called *adjuvant chemotherapy.* For bladder cancer, chemotherapy is sometimes given before surgery to try to improve results or to preserve the bladder. Chemotherapy given in this manner is called *neoadjuvant chemotherapy.* Neoadjuvant chemotherapy is being carefully studied in a clinical trial sponsored by the National Cancer Institute.

Radiation therapy uses high-energy X rays to kill cancer cells and shrink tumors. Radiation may come from a machine outside the body (external-beam radiation therapy) or from putting materials that produce radiation (radioisotopes) through thin plastic tubes in the area where the cancer cells are found (internal radiation therapy).

Biological therapy tries to get the patient's body to fight cancer. It uses materials made by the body or made in a laboratory to boost, direct, or restore the body's natural defenses against disease. Biological therapy is sometimes called biological response modifier (BRM) therapy or immunotherapy.

Photodynamic therapy is a new type of treatment that uses special drugs and light to kill cancer cells. A drug that makes cancer cells more sensitive to light is put into the bladder, and a special light is used to shine on the bladder. This therapy is being studied for early stages of bladder cancer.

Treatment of cancer of the bladder depends on the stage of the disease, the type of disease, and the patient's age and overall condition. The patient may receive treatment that is considered standard based on its effectiveness in a number of patients in past studies, or may choose to go into a clinical trial. Not all patients are cured with standard therapy, and some standard treatments have undesirable side effects. Clinical trials are designed to find better ways to treat cancer patients and are based on the most up-to-date information. Clinical trials are taking place in most parts of the country for most stages of bladder cancer. For more information, call the Cancer Information Service at 1-800-4-CANCER.

TREATMENT BY STAGE

STAGE 0

Treatment may be one of the following:
1. Removal of the cancer using a cystoscope inserted through the urethra to cut out the tumor and burn away any remaining cancer cells (transurethral resection with fulguration).
2. Transurethral resection with fulguration followed by intravesical chemotherapy or biological therapy.
3. Surgery to remove part of the bladder (segmental cystectomy).
4. Intravesical chemotherapy or intravesical biological therapy alone. Clinical trials are evaluating new agents to be given this way.
5. Surgery to remove the whole bladder and organs around it (radical cystectomy).
6. A clinical trial of photodynamic therapy.

STAGE I

Treatment may be one of the following:
1. Removal of the cancer using a cystoscope inserted through the urethra to cut out the tumor and burn away any remaining cancer cells (transurethral resection with fulguration).
2. Transurethral resection and fulguration followed by intravesical chemotherapy or biological therapy.
3. Surgery to remove part of the bladder (segmental cystectomy).
4. Internal radiation therapy with or without external-beam radiation therapy.

5. Intravesical chemotherapy or biological therapy alone.
6. External-beam radiation therapy.
7. Surgery to remove the whole bladder and organs around it (radical cystectomy).

STAGE II   Treatment may be one of the following:

1. Removal of the cancer using a cystoscope inserted through the urethra to cut out the tumor and burn away any remaining cancer cells (transurethral resection with fulguration).
2. Surgery to remove part of the bladder (segmental cystectomy).
3. Surgery to remove the whole bladder and the organs around it (radical cystectomy). The lymph nodes in the pelvis may also be removed (lymph node dissection).
4. External-beam radiation followed by radical cystectomy.
5. Surgery to remove part of the bladder (segmental cystectomy).
6. Internal radiation therapy.
7. A clinical trial of systemic chemotherapy before cystectomy (neoadjuvant chemotherapy) or after cystectomy (adjuvant chemotherapy).
8. A clinical trial of chemotherapy and radiotherapy, which allows the patient to retain the bladder.

STAGE III   Treatment may be one of the following:

1. External radiation therapy followed by surgery to remove the whole bladder and the organs around it (radical cystectomy).
2. Radical cystectomy. The lymph nodes in the pelvis may also be removed (pelvic lymph node dissection).
3. External-beam radiation therapy followed by cystectomy or removal of the

cancer using a cystoscope inserted through the urethra to cut out the tumor and burn away any remaining cancer cells (transurethral resection with fulguration).

4. External-beam and internal radiation therapy.

5. Surgery to remove part of the bladder (segmental cystectomy).

6. Internal radiation therapy.

7. A clinical trial of systemic chemotherapy before cystectomy (neoadjuvant chemotherapy) or after cystectomy (adjuvant chemotherapy).

8. A clinical trial of chemotherapy and radiotherapy, which allows the patient to retain the bladder.

STAGE IV

If the stage IV cancer has spread to nearby tissue or lymph nodes but not to other parts of the body, the treatment may be one of the following:

1. Radiation therapy followed by surgery to remove the whole bladder and organs around it (radical cystectomy). Lymph nodes in the pelvis may also be removed (pelvic lymph node dissection).

2. Radical cystectomy and pelvic lymph node dissection.

3. Radical cystectomy.

4. External-beam radiation therapy.

5. Surgery to make a way for the urine to flow out of the body so that it does not go into the bladder (urinary diversion) to reduce symptoms.

6. Surgery to remove the bladder (cystectomy) to relieve symptoms.

7. Systemic chemotherapy by itself or in addition to surgery.

8. A clinical trial of systemic chemother-

apy before cystectomy (neoadjuvant chemotherapy) or after cystectomy (adjuvant chemotherapy).

9. A clinical trial of systemic chemotherapy and radiation therapy to allow the patient to retain the bladder.

If the cancer is found in lymph nodes or other places far away from the bladder, treatment may be one of the following:

1. External-beam radiation therapy.
2. Surgery to make a way for urine to pass out of the body without going through the bladder (urinary diversion), to reduce symptoms.
3. Surgery to remove the bladder (cystectomy) and to make a urinary diversion to reduce symptoms.
4. Systemic chemotherapy alone or in addition to surgery.

RECURRENT   If the cancer comes back only in the bladder, the patient may receive surgery, chemotherapy, biological therapy, or radiation therapy, depending on what treatment he or she previously received. If the cancer comes back following surgery to remove all of the bladder, the patient may receive chemotherapy or may choose to participate in a clinical trial.

To learn more about bladder cancer, call the National Cancer Institute's Cancer Information Service at 1-800-4-CANCER. The Cancer Information Service can also send the following free booklets about bladder cancer:

Research Report: Cancer of the Bladder
What You Need to Know About Bladder Cancer

The following chart summarizes the current facts about bladder cancer.

BLADDER CANCER

STATUS	49,000 new cases in the United States during 1990
	Accounts for approximately 5% of all cancers
INCIDENCE	Increased approximately 12% between 1973 and 1987
MORTALITY	Decreased approximately 23% between 1973 and 1987
KNOWN CAUSE	Tobacco (Blacks in the United States have high smoking rates and substantial lung cancer rates but relatively low bladder cancer rates. Genetic variations in metabolism of smoking-related carcinogens may thus affect individual risk.)
	Various aniline dyes, certain chemicals in rubber
	Chronic irritation caused by schistosomiasis (infection with a parasitic worm)
LIFESTYLE CHANGES TO PREVENT THE CANCER	Stop smoking, even low-tar cigarettes
	Avoid exposure to aniline dyes
	Increase consumption of fruits and leafy vegetables that contain beta-carotene
MEDICAL INTERVENTION	Encourage lifestyle changes above
	Appropriate treatment of schistosomiasis
	Urge patients to avoid certain occupational hazards
RESEARCH FRONTIERS	In a genetic test under development, urine is tested for cells shed from the bladder that have alterations in tumor-suppressor gene p53.

Chapter 14

Non-Hodgkin's Lymphoma

N ON-HODGKIN'S LYMPHOMA IS THE SIXTH MOST COMMON CANCER IN
the United States. About 35,000 new cases occur each year. The
incidence of non-Hodgkin's lymphoma increases from childhood
through age eighty. Because it tends to strike young—the average age
is forty-two—it ranks fourth among all cancers in economic impact in
the United States. Lymphomas are slightly more common in men than
in women and in white than in black individuals. The course of
lymphomas varies from rapidly fatal to very indolent and initially well
tolerated. Patients with inherited immunologic deficiency diseases,
rheumatoid arthritis, lupus erythematosus, or other rheumatic diseases have a predisposition to lymphomas. Also, patients with AIDS
and those on immunosuppressive drugs after kidney transplants have
a higher incidence than others of an aggressive lymphoma associated
with Epstein-Barr virus infection. Exposure to large doses of radiation,
such as atomic bomb fallout or X rays for arthritic diseases of the spine,
causes lymphomas.

In non-Hodgkin's lymphoma, cancer cells are found in the lymph
system. The lymph system is made up of thin, tubelike vessels that
branch, like veins, into all parts of the body. Lymph vessels carry
lymph, a colorless, watery fluid that contains white blood cells called
lymphocytes. Along the network of vessels are groups of small, bean-
shaped organs called lymph nodes. Clusters of lymph nodes are found
in the underarm, pelvis, neck, and abdomen. The lymph nodes make
and store infection-fighting cells. The spleen (an organ in the upper
abdomen that makes lymphocytes and filters old blood cells from the
blood), the thymus (a small organ beneath the sternum), and the

tonsils are also part of the lymph system. Because lymph tissue is present in so many places, non-Hodgkin's lymphoma can start in almost any part of the body. It can also spread to almost any organ or tissue in the body, including the liver, bone marrow, and spleen.

Lymphomas are divided into two general types: Hodgkin's disease and non-Hodgkin's lymphoma. The cancer cells in Hodgkin's disease have unique microscopic features that are not the same as those in non-Hodgkin's lymphoma. Hodgkin's disease has a more limited spread than non-Hodgkin's lymphoma, and the treatment and prognosis are also different.

In children, non-Hodgkin's lymphoma presents different problems and requires different management approaches than those for adults. For more information about the disease in children, call 1-800-4-CAN-CER and request the PDQ information statement on non-Hodgkin's lymphoma in children. The discussion in this chapter concerns non-Hodgkin's lymphoma in adults.

Screening

No screening tests have been developed for non-Hodgkin's lymphoma.

Diagnosis

Like most cancers, non-Hodgkin's lymphoma is treated most successfully when diagnosed early.

Symptoms   The patient should see a physician if any of the following are present for two weeks or longer:
Painless swelling in the lymph nodes of the neck, underarm, or groin
Persistent fever
Feeling of fatigue
Unexplained weight loss of more than 10 percent in a six-month period
Itchy skin and skin rashes
Small lumps in skin
Bone pain
Swelling in some part of abdomen

Physical Examination If the patient has some of these symptoms, the physician will perform a physical examination with particular attention to lymph nodes in the neck, underarms, and groin. The physician will also look for enlargement of the liver and/or spleen and bone tenderness.

Routine Laboratory Tests

Blood tests. Approximately 30 percent of patients will be anemic.

Urine analysis and tests for kidney function

Chest X rays

Electrocardiogram

Special Laboratory Tests

Bone marrow examinations

Studies of levels of various immune globulins in the serum

Biopsy of lymph node and/or possibly liver

Immunologic studies to determine B, T, or other cell of origin of lymphoma

Radionuclide scans of liver, spleen, and bone

Computerized Tomography (CT) scans

Lymphangiogram to detect lymph nodes in the abdomen that are filled with cancerous cells

Although not all of these tests are required for each patient, enough of them must be performed to obtain a specific diagnosis upon which all future therapy will be based.

Stages of Non-Hodgkin's Lymphoma

When non-Hodgkin's lymphoma is diagnosed, the physician will run more tests to find out whether it has spread from where it started to other parts of the body. This is called staging. The physician needs to know the stage of the disease in order to plan treatment.

The physician may determine the stage of the disease from a physical examination, blood tests, and different kinds of X rays. This is called *clinical staging.* In some cases, the physician may need to do an operation called a laparotomy to determine the stage of the cancer. During this operation, the surgeon cuts into the abdomen and examines the organs inside to see whether they contain cancer. The surgeon will cut out (biopsy) small pieces of tissue during the operation and look at them under a microscope to see whether they contain cancer. This type of staging is called *pathological staging.* Pathological staging is usually done only when it is needed to help the physician plan treatment. The stages of non-Hodgkin's lymphoma are named as follows:

STAGE I   Cancer is found in only one lymph node area or in only one area or organ outside the lymph nodes.

STAGE II   Cancer is found in two or more lymph node areas on the same side of the diaphragm (the thin muscle under the lungs that divides the chest from the abdominal cavities) *or* in only one area or organ outside the lymph nodes and in the lymph nodes around it. Other lymph node areas on the same side of the diaphragm may also have cancer.

STAGE III   Cancer is found in the lymph node areas on both sides of the diaphragm. The cancer may also have spread to an area or organ near the lymph node areas and/or to the spleen.

STAGE IV   Cancer has spread in more than one area to an organ or organs outside the lymph system and may or may not be found in the lymph nodes near these organs, *or* has spread to only one organ outside the lymph system but to lymph nodes far away from that organ.

RELAPSED   Cancer has come back after it has been treated. It may come back in the area where it first started or in another part of the body.

Treatment of Non-Hodgkin's Lymphoma

A patient's prognosis and response to treatment are influenced by the type of cancer cell in the lymphoma. Favorable prognostic types include nodular and well-differentiated B-cell lymphomas. Unfavorable prognostic groups include T-cell or lymphoblastic lymphomas. There are about ten different types of non-Hodgkin's lymphoma. Some types spread more quickly than others. The type is determined by how the cancer cells look under a microscope, which is called the histology. The histologies are grouped together, based on how quickly they spread into low-grade, intermediate-grade, or high-grade lymphomas:

Low Grade	Intermediate Grade	High Grade
Small lymphocytic	Follicular large-cell	Immunoblastic
Large cell		
Follicular small-cleaved	Diffuse small-cleaved	Lymphoblastic small
	Diffuse mixed-cell	Burkitt's or
		non-Burkitt's
Follicular mixed-cell noncleaved	Diffuse large-cell	

As previously discussed, surgery is sometimes used to treat non-Hodgkin's lymphoma. Radiation therapy, which uses high-energy X rays to kill cancer cells and shrink tumors, may also be used. Radiation for non-Hodgkin's lymphoma usually comes from a machine outside the body (external-beam radiation therapy). Radiation therapy given to the neck, chest, and lymph nodes under the arms is called *radiation therapy to a mantle field*. Radiation therapy given to the mantle field and to the lymph nodes in the upper abdomen, the spleen, and the lymph nodes in the pelvis is called *total nodal irradiation*. Radiation given to the brain to keep the cancer cells from growing there is called *cranial irradiation*. Radiation therapy may be used alone or in addition to chemotherapy.

Chemotherapy uses drugs to kill cancer cells and shrink tumors. Chemotherapy may be taken by pill, or it may be injected into the body by a needle in a vein or muscle. Chemotherapy is called a systemic treatment because the drugs enter the bloodstream, travel through the body, and can kill cancer cells throughout the body. Chemotherapy may be put into the fluid that surrounds the brain through a needle in the brain or back *(intrathecal chemotherapy)* to treat certain types of non-Hodgkin's lymphoma that spread to the brain.

Bone marrow transplantation is a newer type of treatment that responds to the very high doses of chemotherapy needed to kill resistant lymphoma cells in the body. Such strong chemotherapy also destroys most of the bone marrow in the body. To replace it, bone marrow is taken from the patient's bones before chemotherapy and treated with drugs or other substances to kill any cancer cells. The marrow is then frozen and the patient is given high-dose chemotherapy with or without radiation therapy to destroy all of the remaining cancer cells. The marrow that was taken out is then thawed and given back to the patient through a needle in a vein. This type of transplant is called an *autologous* transplant. If the marrow returned to the patient was taken from a donor, it is called an *allogeneic* transplant.

Treatment for non-Hodgkin's lymphoma depends on the stage of the disease, the histology and grade of the disease, and the patient's age and general health. The patient may receive treatment that is considered standard based on its effectiveness in a number of patients in past studies, or may choose to go into a clinical trial. Not all patients are cured with standard therapy, and some standard treatments may have undesirable side effects. Clinical trials are designed to find better ways to treat cancer patients and are based on the most up-to-date information. Clinical trials are taking place in most parts of the country for most stages of non-Hodgkin's lymphoma. For more information, call the Cancer Information Service at 1-800-4-CANCER.

TREATMENT BY STAGE

STAGE I

LOW GRADE

Treatment depends on whether the disease is above or below the diaphragm. If the cancer is above the diaphragm, treatment may be one of the following:
1. Radiation therapy to the area where the cancer cells are found.
2. Radiation therapy to a mantle field or only to the neck, upper chest, and lymph nodes under the arms.

If the cancer is below the diaphragm, treatment may be one of the following:
1. Radiation therapy to the area where the cancer cells are found.
2. Radiation to the lymph nodes in the abdomen and pelvis.

INTERMEDIATE GRADE

If the patient had clinical staging (determined by examinations), treatment may be one of the following:

1. Chemotherapy plus radiation therapy.
2. Chemotherapy alone.

If the patient had pathological staging (determined by surgery), treatment may be one of the following:

1. Radiation therapy to mantle field (if the cancer is above the diaphragm).
2. Radiation therapy to the abdomen and the pelvis (if the disease is below the diaphragm).
3. Radiation therapy plus chemotherapy.

HIGH GRADE

Treatment depends on the cell type (histology) of the cancer. If the patient has lymphoblastic lymphoma, treatment may be one of the following:

1. Systemic chemotherapy plus intrathecal chemotherapy.
2. Systemic chemotherapy plus intrathecal chemotherapy and cranial irradiation. Radiation therapy is also given to places in the body with large amounts of cancer.

If the patient has immunoblastic lymphoma, he or she will probably be treated as if it were intermediate-grade lymphoma (see the treatment section on intermediate-grade stage I).

If the patient has small noncleaved cell lymphomas, including Burkitt's lymphoma, treatment will probably be chemotherapy.

STAGE II

LOW GRADE

Treatment depends on whether the disease is above or below the diaphragm. If the patient has cancer above the diaphragm, treatment may be one of the following:

1. Radiation therapy to the area where the cancer cells are found.
2. Radiation therapy to a mantle field or

only to the neck, upper chest, and lymph nodes under the arms.

If the patient has cancer below the diaphragm, treatment may be one of the following:

1. Radiation therapy to the area where the cancer cells are found.
2. Radiation therapy to the lymph nodes in the abdomen and pelvis.

INTERMEDIATE GRADE

Treatment may be one of the following:

1. Systemic chemotherapy.
2. Systemic chemotherapy plus radiation therapy to places where large amounts of cancer are found.
3. Radiation therapy alone (in certain patients).
4. If the cancer is found in the digestive tract, surgery plus chemotherapy.

HIGH GRADE

Treatment depends on the cell type (histology) of the cancer. If the patient has lymphoblastic lymphoma, treatment may be one of the following:

1. Systemic chemotherapy plus intrathecal chemotherapy.
2. Systemic chemotherapy plus intrathecal chemotherapy and cranial irradiation. Radiation therapy is also given to places in the body with large amounts of cancer.

If the patient has immunoblastic lymphoma, he or she will probably be treated as if it were intermediate-grade lymphoma (see the treatment section on intermediate-grade stage II).

If the patient has small noncleaved cell lymphoma, including Burkitt's lymphoma, treatment will probably be chemotherapy. The patient may also want to take part in a clinical trial of bone marrow transplantation or other new treatments.

STAGE III

LOW GRADE

Treatment may be one of the following:
1. If the patient does not have symptoms, he or she may not need treatment. The doctor will watch closely so the patient can be treated if symptoms develop.
2. Systemic chemotherapy.
3. A clinical trial of total nodal irradiation plus systemic chemotherapy.

INTERMEDIATE GRADE

Treatment may be one of the following:
1. Systemic chemotherapy.
2. Systemic chemotherapy plus radiation therapy to places where large amounts of cancer are found.
3. A clinical trial of chemotherapy followed by bone marrow transplantation.

HIGH GRADE

Treatment depends on the cell type (histology) of the cancer. If the patient has lymphoblastic lymphoma, treatment may be one of the following:
1. Systemic chemotherapy plus intrathecal chemotherapy.
2. Systemic chemotherapy plus intrathecal chemotherapy and cranial irradiation. Radiation therapy is also given to places in the body with large amounts of cancer.

If the patient has immunoblastic lymphoma, he or she will probably be treated as if it were intermediate-grade lymphoma (see the treatment section on intermediate-grade stage III).

If the patient has small noncleaved cell lymphoma, including Burkitt's lymphoma, treatment will probably be chemotherapy. He or she may also want to take part in a clinical trial of bone marrow transplantation or other new treatments.

STAGE IV

LOW GRADE

Treatment may be one of the following:
1. If the patient does not have symptoms, he or she may not need treatment. The doctor will watch closely so the patient can be treated if symptoms develop.
2. Systemic chemotherapy.
3. A clinical trial or total nodal irradiation plus system chemotherapy.

INTERMEDIATE GRADE

Treatment may be one of the following:
1. Systemic chemotherapy.
2. Systemic chemotherapy plus radiation therapy to places where large amounts of cancer are found.
3. Systemic chemotherapy plus intrathecal chemotherapy and/or cranial irradiation.
4. A clinical trial of chemotherapy followed by bone marrow transplantation.

HIGH GRADE

Treatment depends on the cell type (histology) of the cancer, but may be one of the following:
1. Systemic chemotherapy plus intrathecal chemotherapy.
2. Systemic chemotherapy plus intrathecal chemotherapy and cranial irradiation. Radiation therapy is also given to places in the body with large amounts of cancer.

If the patient has immunoblastic lymphoma, he or she will probably be treated as if it were intermediate-grade lymphoma (see the treatment section on intermediate-grade stage IV).

If the patient has small noncleaved cell lymphoma, including Burkitt's lymphoma, treatment will probably be chemotherapy. The patient may also want to take part in a clinical trial of bone marrow transplantation or other new treatments.

RELAPSED

LOW GRADE

Low-grade lymphomas often come back after they have been treated. Sometimes the lymphoma will come back as a different cell type (histology), most commonly as an intermediate-grade lymphoma. If this is the case, see the treatment section for recurrent intermediate-grade non-Hodgkin's lymphoma. If the lymphoma comes back and is still a low-grade lymphoma, the treatment may be one of the following:
1. Radiation therapy.
2. Systemic chemotherapy.
3. A clinical trial of bone marrow transplantation.

INTERMEDIATE GRADE

Treatment may be one of the following:
1. Systemic chemotherapy.
2. A clinical trial of chemotherapy followed by bone marrow transplantation.

HIGH GRADE

Treatment may be a clinical trial of bone marrow transplantation or other new treatments.

To learn more about non-Hodgkin's lymphoma, call the National Cancer Institute's Cancer Information Service at 1-800-4-CANCER. The Cancer Information Service can also send the following free booklets about non-Hodgkin's lymphoma:

Research Report: Hodgkin's Disease and the Non-Hodgkin's Lymphomas
What You Need to Know About Non-Hodgkin's Lymphomas

The following chart summarizes the current facts about non-Hodgkin's lymphoma.

NON-HODGKIN'S LYMPHOMA

STATUS	35,600 new cases in the United States during 1990.
	Accounts for approximately 3% of all cancers.
INCIDENCE	Increased approximately 51% between 1973 and 1987. Improved diagnostic procedures may be part of the reason for this increase; some contribution to the increase comes from patients infected with HIV.
MORTALITY	Increased approximately 22% between 1973 and 1987.
KNOWN CAUSES	Human Immunodeficiency Virus (HIV) and HTLV-I.
	A lymphomalike disease is caused by dilantin, a drug used to control seizures.
	Although HIV is associated with non-Hodgkin's lymphoma, it accounts for only a small number of cases, mostly in younger age groups.
	Use of immunosuppressive drugs along with infection with Epstein-Barr Virus (EBV).
	X-ray therapy for arthritis of spine and fallout from atomic bombs.
LIFESTYLE CHANGES TO PREVENT THE CANCER	Avoid infection with HIV and HTLV-1.
MEDICAL INTERVENTION	Institute measures to reduce the AIDS epidemic and the spread of HTLV-1.
	Monitor use of immunosuppressive drugs and therapeutic X rays
RESEARCH FRONTIERS	The origins of two types of lymphoma—Burkitt's lymphoma and follicular lymphoma—have been pinpointed to activation of two protooncogenes, caused by translocation of the two genes to the vicinity of active immunoglobulin genes (see

chapter 3). In Burkitt's lymphoma, the *myc* protooncogene on chromosome 8 is activated, after translocation, by immunoglobulin genes on chromosomes 2, 14, or 22. Such activation of the *myc* gene transforms the normal cell into a lymphoma cell.

In follicular lymphoma, the *bcl*-2 protooncogene on chromosome 18, following translocation, falls under the influence of the active immunoglobulin gene on chromosome 14 and transforms the normal cell into a lymphoma cell. Alterations in *bcl*-6 gene have been detected in about one-third of diffuse large-cell lymphomas.

These cytogenetic changes can be looked for and will aid in specific diagnoses.

Chapter 15

Uterine Cancer

CANCERS OCCUR IN ALL THE ORGANS OF THE FEMALE REPRODUCTIVE tract: the vulva, vagina, cervix (neck of the uterus), uterus (the body of the uterus, or its lining, the endometrium), ovaries, and fallopian tubes. Cancer in each of these sites is associated with distinct symptoms and is diagnosed and treated differently. Of these, cancer of the endometrium or lining of the uterus is the most common, with an estimated 46,500 new cases diagnosed in 1990. This represents about 9 percent of all cancers that affect women and about 48 percent of all female genital cancers.

Approximately 55 to 60 percent of uterine, or endometrial, cancers occur in women between the ages of fifty-five and seventy. Fortunately, about 78 percent of them are diagnosed when they are still localized in the uterus, and therefore they are usually curable. Uterine cancer is more frequent in Jewish women and in women with few or no children. It does not tend to run in families. Although the most common type of uterine cancer is adenocarcinoma, other types, such as squamous-cell cancers, can occur. Postmenopausal women who have taken replacement estrogens are at increased risk of developing uterine cancer, unless the estrogens are taken along with progesterone.

Screening

Because cancer of the endometrium begins inside the uterus, it does not usually show up on the Papanicolaou test, or Pap smear. No useful screening tests for endometrial cancer are currently available.

Diagnosis

Symptoms The first symptom of uterine cancer is abnormal vaginal bleeding of fresh blood or a watery bloody discharge in a postmenopausal woman. In fact, 70 to 75 percent of the women who develop uterine cancer are postmenopausal, so vaginal bleeding or discharge is an alarming symptom that should immediately be recognized as abnormal by the woman and should cause her to seek medical help. Fortunately, these symptoms are sometimes caused by nonmalignant fibromas or other disorders, but it is important to seek a definitive diagnosis. In women with some blockage of the cervical canal, a collection of fluid may occur in the uterus and is always suggestive of uterine cancer.

Other symptoms include difficult or painful urination, pain during intercourse, and pain in the pelvic area.

Physical Examination After a routine health history, the physician will do a physical examination including an internal (pelvic) examination, during which he or she will feel for any lumps or changes in the shape of the uterus. The physician will then do a Pap test using a piece of cotton and a brush or a small wooden stick to scrape gently the outside of the cervix (opening of the uterus) and vagina to pick up cells. Of note, while Pap smears are about 97 percent effective in diagnosing carcinomas of the cervix, they are less than 50 percent accurate in diagnosing cancer of the endometrium.

Routine Laboratory Tests

Routine blood tests and urine analysis for general health status, kidney function, and infections in the urinary tract

Chest X ray to visualize pneumonia

Electrocardiogram to evaluate heart function

Other blood tests, liver function tests

Pap smear

Special Laboratory Tests To specifically diagnose the cancer and "stage" it—that is, to determine whether it has spread to other organs, such as the bladder or rectum.

ASPIRATION CURETTAGE OF ENDOMETRIUM In this test a small tube attached to a syringe is inserted through the cervical opening into the uterine cavity, and small fragments of the lining are sucked or aspirated into the syringe. This tissue is then checked for cancer cells.

DILATATION AND CURETTAGE OF THE ENDOMETRIUM For this test

the patient is anesthetized and the gynecologist stretches the opening of the cervix with a spoon-shaped instrument. A scraping instrument called a curette is then inserted into the uterus, and small fragments of the uterine wall are scraped gently to remove any growths. The fragments of tissue obtained are checked by a pathologist for cancer.

OTHER TESTS AS DEEMED NECESSARY   A barium enema, observation of the bladder *(cystoscopy)*, and observation of the lower colon *(proctosigmoidoscopy)*, as well as CT and MRI scans, may be helpful in the complete diagnostic workup of a woman with uterine cancer. All seek evidence that a uterine tumor is impinging on the bladder or colon.

Although not all of these tests are required for each patient, enough of them must be performed to obtain a specific diagnosis upon which all future therapy will be based.

Stages of Uterine Cancer

As described, when cancer of the endometrium has been diagnosed, more tests will be done to find out whether it has spread from the endometrium to other parts of the body. The physician needs to know the stage of the disease in order to plan treatment. The stages of uterine cancer are named as follows:

STAGE 0	Or carcinoma *in situ*, a very early cancer found inside the uterus only, and in only the surface layer of the endometrium.
STAGE I	Cancer is found only in the main part of the uterus (not in the cervix).
STAGE II	Cancer cells have spread to the cervix.
STAGE III	Cancer cells have spread outside the uterus but have not spread outside the pelvis.
STAGE IV	Cancer cells have spread beyond the pelvis, to other body parts or into the lining of the bladder or rectum.
RECURRENT	Cancer has come back after it has been treated.

Treatment of Uterine Cancer

As with most cancers, uterine cancer can be treated successfully if diagnosed early. The choice of treatment depends upon the stage of the disease and, if diagnosed early, also upon whether female hormones affect the growth of cancer cells. There are treatments for all patients with cancer of the endometrium. Four kinds of treatment are used: surgery, radiation therapy, chemotherapy, and hormone therapy.

Surgery is the most common treatment for cancer of the endometrium. The physician may take out the cancer using one of the following operations:

Total abdominal hysterectomy and bilateral salpingo-oophorectomy, taking out the uterus, fallopian tubes, and ovaries through an incision in the abdomen. Lymph nodes in the pelvis may also be taken out (lymph node dissection).
Radical hysterectomy, taking out the cervix, uterus, fallopian tubes, ovaries, and part of the vagina. Lymph nodes in the area may also be taken out.

Radiation therapy uses high-dose X rays to kill cancer cells and shrink tumors. Radiation may come from a machine outside the body (external radiation) or from putting materials that produce radiation (radioisotopes) through thin plastic tubes into the area where the cancer cells are found (internal radiation). Radiation may be used alone or before or after surgery.

Chemotherapy uses drugs to kill cancer cells. Chemotherapy may be taken by pill or may be put into the body intravenously. Chemotherapy is called a systemic treatment because the drugs enter the bloodstream, travel through the body, and can kill cancer cells outside the uterus.

Hormone therapy uses hormones, usually taken by pill, to kill cancer cells.

Treatment for cancer of the endometrium depends on the stage of the disease, the type of disease, and the patient's age and overall condition. The patient may receive treatment that is considered standard based on its effectiveness in a number of patients in past studies, or she may choose to go into a clinical trial. Not all patients are cured with standard therapy, and some standard treatments may have undesirable side effects. Clinical trials are designed to find better ways to treat cancer patients and are based on the most up-to-date information. Clinical trials are taking place in most parts of the country for most stages of cancer of the endometrium. For more information, call the Cancer Information Service at 1-800-4-CANCER.

TREATMENT BY STAGE

STAGE 0   Treatment may be one of the following:
1. Dilatation and curettage (D & C) followed by hormone therapy. The physician may tell the patient not to take any more medicine that contains estrogen.
2. Hysterectomy.

STAGE I   Treatment may be one of the following:
1. Total abdominal hysterectomy and bilateral salpingo-oophorectomy, with removal of some of the lymph nodes in the pelvis and abdomen to test for cancer.
2. Total abdominal hysterectomy and bilateral salpingo-oophorectomy, with removal of some of the lymph nodes in the pelvis and abdomen to test for cancer, followed by radiation therapy to the pelvis.
3. Clinical trials of radiation and/or chemotherapy following surgery.
4. Radiation therapy alone for selected patients.

STAGE II   Treatment may be one of the following:
1. Internal- and external-beam radiation therapy followed by total abdominal hysterectomy and bilateral salpingo-oophorectomy. Some of the lymph nodes in the pelvis and abdomen are also removed to see whether they are cancerous.
2. Total abdominal hysterectomy, bilat-

eral salpingo-oophorectomy, and removal of some of the lymph nodes in the pelvis and abdomen to see whether they contain cancer, followed by radiation therapy.

3. Radical hysterectomy. Lymph nodes in the area may also be taken out (lymph node dissection).

STAGE III   Treatment may be one of the following:

1. Radical hysterectomy. Lymph nodes in the area may also be taken out (lymph node dissection). Surgery is usually followed by radiation therapy.
2. Internal- and external-beam radiation therapy.
3. Hormone therapy.

STAGE IV   Treatment may be one of the following:

1. Internal- and external-beam radiation therapy.
2. Hormone therapy.
3. Clinical trials of chemotherapy.

RECURRENT   If the cancer has recurred, treatment may be one of the following:

1. Radiation therapy to relieve symptoms such as pain, nausea, and abnormal bowel functions.
2. Hormone therapy.
3. Clinical trials of chemotherapy.

To learn more about cancer of the endometrium, call the National Cancer Institute's Cancer Information Service at 1-800-4-CANCER. The Cancer Information Service can also send the following free booklets on uterine cancer:

What You Need to Know About Cancer of the Uterus
Research Report: Cancer of the Uterus

The following chart summarizes the current facts about uterine cancer.

UTERINE CANCER

STATUS	46,500 new cases in the United States during 1990
INCIDENCE	Decreased approximately 26% between 1973 and 1987
MORTALITY	Decreased approximately 20% between 1973 and 1987
KNOWN CAUSE	The female hormone estrogen
LIFESTYLE CHANGES TO PREVENT THE CANCER	Add progesterone to estrogen in estrogen-replacement therapy for postmenopausal women
MEDICAL INTERVENTION	Avoid the use of high-dose estrogen without progesterone in postmenopausal women
	Oral contraceptives may reduce risk of uterine cancer
RESEARCH FRONTIERS	All patients with advanced and recurrent disease are being considered as candidates for clinical trials of new chemotherapeutic agents.

Chapter 16

Cancers of the Oral Cavity, Lip, and Pharynx

CIGARETTE SMOKING AS WELL AS CIGAR AND PIPE SMOKING ARE MAJOR causes of cancers of the oral cavity, including the cheeks (buccal mucosa), tongue, floor of the mouth, gums (gingiva), and pharynx. Heavy alcohol consumption increases the risk of these cancers, especially in conjunction with smoking. Smokers who consume seven or more ounces of alcohol daily have a fivefold increase in risk for oral cancer, even if they smoke fewer than ten cigarettes a day. The risk rises twenty-four times if they smoke more than a pack a day. Squamous-cell cancer of the oral cavity, associated with use of tobacco and alcohol, occurs mostly in men between the ages of sixty and seventy.

Cancer of the oral cavity and pharynx is the eighth most common cancer. In 1990 over 30,000 new cases were diagnosed in the United States, accounting for 3 percent of new cancers that year. Although the incidence of these cancers remained stable from 1973 to 1987 (a decrease of 1.3 percent), the mortality decreased 16 percent due to more effective treatment. The five-year survival rate is 52 percent, the same as the average survival rate for all cancers.

Early stages of these tumors usually cause no pain or other symptoms. Nonetheless, they are easy to detect: Any ulcer of the oral mucosa that does not improve after one week of treatment should be considered malignant until proven otherwise. Many cancers of the mouth are first detected by dentists.

While most tumors of the lip are benign, lip cancer does occur, usually in men between the ages of sixty and seventy. It appears mainly on the lower lip, most commonly in smokers who hold a cigarette or pipe in one location. Chapping and prolonged exposure to sunlight, especially in fair-skinned individuals, are also factors causing lip cancer.

Screening

The National Cancer Institute's working guidelines for oral cavity cancer recommend that "oral examination including palpation of the tongue, floor of the mouth, salivary glands and lymph nodes be performed as part of a periodic health examination," and that "special attention should be given to those at high risk due to tobacco and alcoholism."

Diagnosis

The earliest cancers cause no symptoms. They are red, slightly elevated sores with indistinct margins. White patches *(leukoplakia)* on the lip, tongue, or mouth—called smoker's patches or smoker's tongue—are not cancerous at first, but 100 percent of them can develop into cancer if continually irritated by smoking.

Symptoms As the cancer progresses, the patient can often feel a lump in the mouth with the tongue. Sometimes a sore spot can be felt while eating or drinking, or one may have an ulceration of the lips, tongue, or other area inside the mouth that does not heal within two weeks. Dentures may no longer fit well. Advanced cancers cause pain, bleeding, foul breath, loose teeth, and changes in speech.

Physical Examination After taking a health history, the physician will examine the mouth and feel for enlarged lymph nodes in the neck. Any suspicious area will be biopsied or removed entirely.

Routine Laboratory Tests
Blood tests
Urine analysis
Chest X ray
Electrocardiogram

Special Laboratory Tests

  X-ray examination of the lower jaw
  Computerized Tomography (CT) scan to determine extent of local
    spread and invasion of bone
  Excision of small lesions, incision or punch biopsy of large lesions

Although not all of these tests are required for each patient, enough
of them must be performed to obtain a specific diagnosis upon which
all future therapy will be based.

Stages of Oral Cavity and Lip Cancer

When cancer of the lip or oral cavity is found, the tests just described
will be done to find out whether cancer cells have spread to other parts
of the body. This is called staging. The physician needs to know the
stage of the disease in order to plan treatment. The stages of oral cavity
and lip cancer are named as follows:

STAGE I   Cancer is no more than 2 centimeters
                     (about 1 inch) and has not spread to lymph
                     nodes in the area.

STAGE II   Cancer is more than 2 centimeters but less
                     than 4 centimeters (less than 2 inches) and
                     has not spread to lymph nodes in the area.

STAGE III   Cancer is more than 4 centimeters, *or* the
                     cancer is any size but has spread to only
                     one lymph node on the same side of the
                     neck as the cancer. The lymph node that
                     contains cancer measures no more than 3
                     centimeters (just over 1 inch).

STAGE IV   Any of the following may be true:

                     Cancer has spread to tissues around the lip
                       and oral cavity.

                     The lymph nodes in the area may or may
                       not contain cancer.

The cancer is any size and has spread to more than one lymph node on the same side of the neck as the cancer, to lymph nodes on one or both sides of the neck, or to any lymph node that measures more than 6 centimeters (over 2 inches).

The cancer has spread to other parts of the body.

RECURRENT   The cancer has come back after it has been treated. It may come back in the lip and oral cavity or in another part of the body.

Treatment of Oral Cavity and Lip Cancer

Surgery and radiation therapy are used to treat all patients with cancer of the lip and oral cavity. Chemotherapy is being tested in clinical trials. The surgeon may remove the cancer, some of the surrounding healthy tissue, and maybe the lymph nodes in the neck (lymph node dissection). A new type of surgery called *micrographic surgery* is being tested in clinical trials for early cancers of the lip and oral cavity. During this surgery, the surgeon removes the cancer and then uses a microscope to examine the area to make sure there are no cancer cells left. As little normal tissue as possible is removed.

Radiation therapy uses high-energy X rays to kill cancer cells and shrink tumors. Radiation may come from a machine outside the body (external-beam radiation therapy) or from putting materials that produce radiation (radioisotopes) through thin plastic tubes or needles into the area where the cancer cells are found (internal radiation therapy).

If the surgeon removes all the cancer that can be seen at the time of the operation, the patient may be given chemotherapy after surgery to kill any cancer cells that are left. If given after an operation to a person who has no cancer cells that can be seen, it is called *adjuvant chemotherapy*. If given before surgery to try to shrink the cancer so that it can be removed, it is called *neoadjuvant chemotherapy*.

Hyperthermia is a new treatment being tested on certain patients. It uses a special machine to heat the body for a certain period of time to kill cancer cells. Because cancer cells are often more sensitive to heat than normal cells, the cancer cells die and the cancer shrinks.

Because our lips and mouths help us eat and talk, people with cancer in this region may need special help adjusting to the side effects of the cancer and its treatment. The physician will consult with several kinds of specialists who can help determine the best treatment for the patient. Trained medical staff can also help the patient recover from treatment and adjust to new ways of eating and talking. The patient may need plastic surgery or help in learning to eat and speak if a large part of the lip or mouth is removed.

Treatment for cancer of the lip and oral cavity depends on where the cancer is, what stage it is in, and the patient's age and overall health. The patient may receive treatment that is considered standard based on its effectiveness in a number of patients in past studies, or may choose to go into a clinical trial. Not all patients are cured with standard therapy, and some standard treatments have undesirable side effects. Clinical trials are designed to find better ways to treat cancer patients and are based on the most up-to-date information. Clinical trials are taking place in many parts of the country for patients with cancer of the lip and oral cavity. For more information, call the Cancer Information Service at 1-800-4-CANCER.

TREATMENT BY STAGE

STAGE I ORAL CAVITY AND LIP CANCER

Treatment depends on where the cancer is. If the cancer is in the buccal mucosa (lining of the cheeks), floor of the mouth, lower and upper gum, or hard palate, the treatment may be one of the following:

1. Surgery.
2. Radiation therapy.

TONGUE CANCER

If the cancer is in the tongue, treatment may be one of the following:

1. Surgery.
2. Surgery followed by radiation therapy to the neck.
3. Radiation therapy to the mouth and the neck.

RETROMOLAR TRIGONE CANCER

If the cancer is in the small area behind the wisdom teeth (*retromolar trigone*), treatment may be one of the following:

1. Surgery to remove part of the jawbone.
2. Radiation therapy followed (if needed) by surgery.

For all stage I oral cavity and lip cancers, clinical trials are testing micrographic surgery followed by radiation therapy.

STAGE II ORAL CAVITY AND LIP CANCER

Treatment depends on where the cancer is. If the cancer is in the lip, treatment may be one of the following:
1. Surgery.
2. Internal and/or external radiation therapy.

TONGUE CANCER

Treatment may be one of the following:
1. Radiation therapy.
2. Surgery and radiation therapy.

BUCCAL MUCOSA CANCER

Treatment may be one of the following:
1. Radiation therapy.
2. Surgery.
3. Surgery plus radiation therapy.

CANCER OF THE FLOOR OF THE MOUTH

Treatment may be one of the following:
1. Surgery.
2. Radiation therapy.
3. Surgery followed by internal or external-beam radiation therapy.

LOWER GUM CANCER

Treatment may be one of the following:
1. Surgery.
2. Radiation therapy.

RETROMOLAR TRIGONE CANCER

Treatment may be one of the following:
1. Surgery to remove part of the jawbone.
2. Radiation therapy followed (if needed) by surgery.

UPPER GUM OR HARD PALATE CANCER

Treatment will probably be surgery followed by radiation therapy. For all stage II oral cavity and lip cancers, clinical trials are testing micrographic surgery followed by radiation therapy.

STAGE III ORAL CAVITY AND LIP CANCER

Treatment depends on where the cancer is. In addition to the treatments listed below, the patient will probably have radiation therapy to the neck, with or without surgery to remove lymph nodes in the neck (lymph node dissection).

LIP CANCER

Treatment may be one of the following:

1. Surgery to remove the cancer plus internal or external radiation therapy.
2. A clinical trial of chemotherapy followed by surgery or radiation therapy.
3. A clinical trial of surgery followed by chemotherapy.
4. A clinical trial of surgery, radiation therapy, and chemotherapy.

TONGUE CANCER

Treatment may be one of the following:

1. External beam with or without internal radiation therapy.
2. Surgery followed by radiation therapy.

BUCCAL MUCOSA CANCER

Treatment may be one of the following:

1. Surgery to remove the cancer and the tissue around it.
2. Radiation therapy.
3. Surgery plus radiation therapy.
4. A clinical trial of chemotherapy followed by surgery or radiation therapy.

5. A clinical trial of surgery followed by chemotherapy.

6. A clinical trial of surgery, radiation therapy, and chemotherapy.

Cancer of the Floor of the Mouth

Treatment may be one of the following:

1. Surgery to remove the cancer and lymph nodes in the neck. Part of the jawbone may also be removed if necessary.

2. External-beam radiation therapy, with or without internal radiation therapy.

3. A clinical trial of chemotherapy followed by surgery or radiation therapy.

4. A clinical trial of surgery followed by chemotherapy.

5. A clinical trial of surgery, radiation therapy, and chemotherapy.

Lower Gum Cancer

Treatment will probably be radiation therapy given before or after surgery to remove the cancer.

Retromolar Trigone Cancer

Treatment may be one of the following:

1. Surgery followed by radiation therapy.

2. A clinical trial of chemotherapy followed by surgery or radiation therapy.

3. A clinical trial of surgery followed by chemotherapy.

4. A clinical trial of surgery, radiation therapy, and chemotherapy.

Upper Gum or Hard Palate Cancer

Treatment may be one of the following:

1. Radiation therapy.

2. Surgery plus radiation therapy.

For all stage III oral cavity and lip cancers, clinical trials are testing micrographic surgery followed by radiation therapy.

STAGE IV ORAL CAVITY AND LIP CANCER
Treatment depends on where the cancer is. In addition to the treatments described for stage III, the patient will probably have radiation therapy to the neck, with or without surgery to remove lymph nodes in the neck (lymph node dissection).

RECURRENT ORAL CAVITY AND LIP CANCER
Treatment depends on the type of treatment the patient has already had. If the patient has had radiation therapy, surgery may be used when the cancer recurs. If the patient has had surgery, he or she may have more surgery, radiation therapy, or both. The patient may want to consider taking part in a clinical trial of chemotherapy or hyperthermia.

To learn more about cancer of the oral cavity and lip, call the National Cancer Institute's Cancer Information Service at 1-800-4-CANCER.

Cancer of the pharynx is another common oral cancer. The *pharynx* is a hollow tube about 5 inches long that connects the nose and mouth to the esophagus. The *oropharynx* is the middle part of the throat that includes the soft palate (back of the mouth), the base of the tongue, and the tonsils. The *hypopharynx* is the bottom part of the throat. The *nasopharynx* is behind the nose; it is the upper part of the throat.

Cancers in these regions of the pharynx start in the cells that line the pharynx, called squamous cells. The various features of these cancers such as diagnosis and treatment are similar to oral cavity and lip cancer. Therefore, only those of the oropharynx are described here. The most common site for this cancer is on the tonsil.

Screening

No screening tests are currently available for cancer of the pharynx other than those of the mouth and lymph nodes previously described.

Diagnosis

Symptoms   The earliest symptom of cancer of the pharynx is a mild sore throat that is localized to one side. This symptom is rather specific for cancer, since infectious sore throat occurs on both sides. The patient with cancer can often point to the painful site with one finger, whereas the patient with an infectious sore throat can not. The cancer may appear as a velvety red patch or open sore, causing only mild pain. In more advanced cases, the patient may have difficulty swallowing or breathing, may have the sensation of a foreign body, a headache, an earache, blood-stained saliva, regurgitation of food and liquid, and voice changes. A lump or mass in the neck may be the initial sign.

Physical Examination   After eliciting a health history, the physician will make a complete physical examination to detect any lesions in the lining of the throat or tonsils or any enlarged lymph nodes in the neck. The physician may also use a laryngoscope to observe the lower parts of the throat.

Routine Laboratory Tests   The same as those obtained for oral cancers.

Special Laboratory Tests

Computerized Tomography (CT) scans are useful in determining any invasion of the cancer into adjacent issues and lymph node metastases. Such scans should be done before biopsy.

Some lesions in the oropharynx can be biopsied in the physician's office under local anesthesia.

Stages of Cancer of the Oropharynx

When cancer of the oropharynx is diagnosed, the tests just described will be done to find out whether cancer cells have spread to other parts of the body. This is called staging. The physician needs to know the stage of the disease in order to plan treatment. The stages of cancer of the oropharynx are named as follows:

STAGE I	Cancer is no more than 2 centimeters (about 1 inch) and has not spread to lymph nodes in the area.
STAGE II	Cancer is more than 2 centimeters but less than 4 centimeters (less than 2 inches), and has not spread to lymph nodes in the area.
STAGE III	Either of the following may be true:
	Cancer is more than 4 centimeters.
	Cancer is any size but has spread to only one lymph node on the same side of the neck as the cancer. The lymph node that contains the cancer measures no more than 3 centimeters (just over 1 inch).
STAGE IV	Any of the following may be true:
	Cancer has spread to tissue around the oropharynx. The lymph nodes in the area may or may not contain cancer.
	Cancer is any size and has spread to more than one lymph node on the same side of the neck as the cancer, to lymph nodes or one or both sides of the neck, or to any lymph node that measures more than 6 centimeters (over 2 inches).
	Cancer has spread to other parts of the body.
RECURRENT	Cancer has come back after it has been treated. It may come back in the oropharynx or in another part of the body.

Treatment of Cancer of the Oropharynx

Three kinds of treatment may be used for patients with cancer of the oropharynx: surgery, radiation therapy, and chemotherapy. Hyperthermia (warming the body to kill cancer cells) is being tested in clinical trials. In surgery, the surgeon may remove the cancer and some of the healthy tissue around the cancer. If cancer has spread to lymph nodes, the lymph nodes will be removed (lymph node dissection). A new type of surgery called *micrographic surgery* is being tested in clinical trials for early cancers of the oropharynx. Micrographic surgery removes the cancer and as little normal tissue as possible. During this surgery, the surgeon removes the cancer, then uses a microscope to examine the cancerous area to make sure there are no remaining cancer cells.

Radiation therapy uses high-energy X rays to kill cancer cells and shrink tumors. Radiation may come from a machine outside the body (external-beam radiation therapy) or from putting materials that produce radiation (radioisotopes) through thin plastic tubes into the area where the cancer cells are found (internal radiation therapy). Giving drugs with radiation therapy to make the cancer cells more sensitive to radiation (radiosensitization) is being tested in clinical trials.

Chemotherapy uses drugs to kill cancer cells. Chemotherapy may be taken by pill or may be put into the body intravenously. Chemotherapy is called a systemic treatment because the drugs enter the bloodstream, travel through the body, and can kill cancer cells throughout the body.

Hyperthermia uses a special machine to heat the body for a certain period of time to kill cancer cells. Because cancer cells are often more sensitive to heat than normal cells, the cancer cells die and the cancer shrinks.

Because the oropharynx helps us breathe, eat, and talk, the patient with cancer of the oropharynx may need special help adjusting to the side effects of the cancer and its treatment. The physician will consult with several specialists who can help determine the best treatment for the patient. Trained medical staff can also help the patient recover from treatment and adjust to new ways of eating and talking. The patient may also need plastic surgery or help in learning to eat and speak again if a large part of the oropharynx is taken out.

Treatment for cancer of the oropharynx depends on where the

cancer is, what stage it is in, and the patient's age and overall health. The patient may receive treatment that is considered standard based on its effectiveness in a number of patients in past studies, or may choose to go into a clinical trial. Not all patients are cured with standard therapy, and some standard treatments may have undesirable side effects. Clinical trials are designed to find better ways to treat cancer and are based on the most up-to-date information. Clinical trials are taking place in many parts of the country for patients with cancer of the oropharynx. For more information, call the Cancer Information Service at 1-800-4-CANCER.

TREATMENT BY STAGE

STAGE I OR STAGE II
Treatment may be one of the following:
1. Surgery to remove the cancer.
2. Radiation therapy. Clinical trials are testing new ways of giving radiation therapy.
3. A clinical trial of microsurgery followed by radiation therapy.

STAGE III
Treatment may be one of the following:
1. Surgery to remove the cancer followed by radiation therapy.
2. A clinical trial of chemotherapy followed by surgery or radiation therapy.
3. A clinical trial of radiation therapy given with drugs to make the cancer cells more sensitive to radiation therapy (radiosensitizers).
4. A clinical trial of new ways of giving radiation therapy.
5. A clinical trial of microsurgery followed by radiation therapy.

STAGE IV
If the cancer can be removed by surgery, treatment may be one of the following:
1. Surgery to remove the cancer followed by radiation therapy.
2. A clinical trial of radiation therapy given with chemotherapy or drugs to

make the cancer cells more sensitive to radiation therapy (radiosensitizers).

3. A clinical trial of new ways of giving radiation therapy.

4. A clinical trial of microsurgery followed by radiation therapy.

If the cancer cannot be removed by surgery, treatment may be one of the following:

1. Radiation therapy. Clinical trials are testing new ways of giving radiation therapy.

2. A clinical trial of chemotherapy followed by surgery or radiation therapy.

3. A clinical trial of radiation therapy given with chemotherapy or with drugs to make the cancer cells more sensitive to radiation therapy (radiosensitizers).

4. A clinical trial of hyperthermia plus radiation therapy.

RECURRENT   Treatment may be one of the following:

1. Surgery to remove the cancer.

2. Radiation therapy.

3. A clinical trial of chemotherapy.

4. A clinical trial of hyperthermia plus radiation therapy.

To learn more about cancer of the oropharynx, call the National Cancer Institute's Cancer Information Service at 1-800-4-CANCER.

The following chart summarizes the current facts about cancer of the oral cavity, lip, and pharynx.

CANCERS OF THE ORAL CAVITY, LIP, AND PHARYNX

STATUS	30,500 new cases in the United States during 1990
	Accounts for approximately 3% of all cancers
INCIDENCE	Decreased 1.3% between 1973 and 1987
MORTALITY	Decreased approximately 16% between 1973 and 1987, probably due to improved treatment
	5-year survival rate is 52%.
KNOWN CAUSES	Tobacco and alcohol have symbiotic effect, related to the number of cigarettes smoked and ounces of alcohol consumed
LIFESTYLE CHANGES TO PREVENT THE CANCER	Stop smoking even low-tar cigarettes and pipes
	Stop use of smokeless tobacco, snuff, and chewing tobacco
	Discontinue heavy use of both tobacco and alcohol
	Increase consumption of fruits and leafy vegetables that contain beta-carotene
MEDICAL INTERVENTION	Encourage lifestyle changes above.
	As part of periodic health examination, include palpation of tongue, floor of mouth, salivary glands, and lymph nodes of the neck.
	Give special attention to those at high risk due to tobacco and alcohol use.
	Advise individuals with fair skin, especially redheads, to avoid prolonged exposure to sunlight, to wear a hat, and to use an antiactinic cream on the lips.

Chapter 17

Cancer of the Pancreas

CANCER OF THE PANCREAS IS A HIGHLY MALIGNANT DISEASE. IT IS THE ninth largest cancer killer in adults in the United States, and very few who develop it are lucky enough to survive. In 1990, over 28,000 new cases were diagnosed in the United States, and of these 25,000 will eventually die of it. Cancer of the pancreas has the lowest five-year survival rate (3 percent) of any cancer. It tends to occur in older people, median age about sixty-nine, and is slightly more common in men than in women (1.7:1.0) and in black men than in white, Spanish, or Chinese. Cigarette smoking has been associated with increased risk of cancer of the pancreas, as has long-term exposure (ten years or more) to industrial chemicals such as benzidine and beta-naphthylamine (DeVita et al. 1989; Henderson et al. 1991). Drinking large amounts of coffee was considered to cause pancreatic cancer in the early 1980s, but follow-up studies did not confirm this association. Alcohol consumption is not associated with this cancer either.

In cancer of the pancreas, cancer cells are found in the tissues of the pancreas. The pancreas is about 6 inches long and is shaped something like a thin pear, wider at one end and narrowing at the other. The pancreas lies behind the stomach, inside a loop formed by part of the small intestine. The broader right end of the pancreas is called the head, the middle section is called the body, and the narrow left end is the tail.

The pancreas has two basic functions. It produces juices that help break down (digest) food, and hormones (such as insulin) that regulate how the body stores and uses food. The area of the pancreas that produces digestive juices is called the *exocrine* pancreas. About 95 percent of pancreatic cancers begin in the exocrine pancreas. The hormone-producing area of the pancreas is called the *endocrine* pancreas. Only about 5 percent of pancreatic cancers start here. This chapter presents information on cancer of the exocrine pancreas. For more information on cancer of the endocrine pancreas (also called islet cell cancer), request the PDQ Patient Information Statement on Islet Cell Carcinoma by calling 1-800-4-CANCER.

Screening

No screening tests are currently available for pancreatic cancer. Advances in monoclonal antibody technology might provide such tests in the future.

Diagnosis

Unfortunately, by the time most patients are diagnosed, the disease has advanced beyond the scope of curative treatment. Cancer of the pancreas is hard to diagnose because the organ is hidden behind the stomach, the small intestine, bile ducts (tubes through which bile, a digestive juice made by the liver, flows from the liver into the small intestine), the gallbladder (the small sac below the liver that stores bile), the liver, and the spleen (the organ that stores red blood cells and filters blood to remove excess blood cells). The signs of pancreatic cancer resemble those of many other illnesses, and there may be no signs in the first stages.

Symptoms   The hallmarks of pancreatic cancer are abdominal pain and unexplained weight loss. At the time of diagnosis, 90 percent of patients have abdominal pain and more than a 10 percent weight loss. Severe upper abdominal pain often radiates to the back. Other symptoms are loss of appetite, intolerance of fatty foods, and yellowing of the skin (jaundice due to blockage of the bile duct).

Physical Examination   After eliciting a health history, the physician will make a complete physical examination to detect any abdominal masses, including enlargement of the liver or spleen, or jaundice.

Routine Laboratory Tests
   Blood Tests
   Urinalysis
   Chest X ray
   Electrocardiogram
Special Laboratory Tests
   Ultrasound test, using sound waves to find tumors, is often done
      first.
   Computerized Tomography (CT scan) may be done if the
      ultrasound is negative or indeterminate.
   Magnetic Resonance Imaging (MRI) may be done as well, to further
      clarify the diagnosis.
   Endoscopic retrograde cholangiopancreatography (ERCP) may also
      be done. During this test, a flexible tube is put down the throat,
      through the stomach, and into the small intestine. The physician
      can see through the tube and inject dye into the drainage tube
      (duct) of the pancreas so that the area can be seen more clearly on
      an X ray. During ERCP, the physician may also put a fine needle
      into the pancreas to take out some cells (biopsy). The cells can
      then be looked at under a microscope to see whether they are
      cancerous.
   Percutaneous transhepatic cholangiography (PTC) is another test
      that can help find cancer of the pancreas. During this test, a thin
      needle is put into the liver through the right side. Dye is injected
      into the bile ducts in the liver so that blockages can be seen on
      X rays.
   Laparotomy surgery may be required to diagnose cancer of the
      pancreas. If this is the case, the surgeon will open the abdomen
      and examine the pancreas and the tissue around it for cancer. If
      cancer is found and it looks like it has not spread to other tissues,
      the surgeon may remove the cancer or relieve blockages caused
      by the tumor.

   Although not all of these tests are required for each patient, enough
of them must be performed to obtain a specific diagnosis upon which
all future therapy will be based.

Stages of Pancreatic Cancer

Once cancer of the pancreas is found, more tests will be done to find out whether the cancer has spread to the surrounding tissues or to other parts of the body. This is called staging. The stages of pancreatic cancer are named as follows:

STAGE I	Cancer is found only in the pancreas itself, or has started to spread only to the tissues next to the pancreas, such as the small intestine, the stomach, or the bile duct.
STAGE II	Cancer has spread to nearby organs, such as the stomach, spleen, or colon, but has not entered the lymph nodes.
STAGE III	Cancer has spread to the lymph nodes near the pancreas. It may or may not have spread to nearby organs.
STAGE IV	Cancer has spread to places far away from the pancreas, such as the liver or lungs.
RECURRENT	Cancer has come back after it has been treated. It may come back in the pancreas or in another part of the body.

Treatment of Pancreatic Cancer

Three kinds of treatment are used for patients with cancer of the pancreas: surgery, radiation therapy, and chemotherapy. The use of biological therapy (using the body's immune system to fight cancer) is being tested. If surgery is chosen, the surgeon may take out the cancer using one of the following operations:

A *Whipple* procedure removes the head of the pancreas, part of the small intestine, and some of the tissues around it. Enough of the pancreas is left to continue making digestive juices and insulin.
Total pancreatectomy takes out the whole pancreas, part of the small intestine, part of the stomach, the bile duct, the gallbladder, the spleen, and most of the lymph nodes in the area.
Distal pancreatectomy takes out only the tail of the pancreas. If the cancer has spread and cannot be removed, the surgeon may do surgery to relieve symptoms. If the cancer is blocking the small

intestine and bile builds up in the gallbladder, the surgeon may do surgery to go around (bypass) all or part of the small intestine. During this operation, the surgeon will cut the gallbladder or bile duct and sew it to the small intestine. This is called *biliary bypass*. Surgery or X-ray procedures may also be done to put in a tube (catheter) to drain bile that has built up in the area. During these procedures, the surgeon may make the catheter drain through a tube to the outside of the body, or the catheter may go around the blocked area and drain the bile to the small intestine. In addition, if the cancer is blocking the flow of food from the stomach, the stomach may be sewn directly to the small intestine so that the patient can continue to eat normally.

Radiation therapy uses high-energy X rays to kill cancer cells and shrink tumors.

Chemotherapy uses drugs to kill cancer cells. Chemotherapy may be taken by pill, or it may be put into the body by a needle in the vein or muscle. Chemotherapy is called a systemic treatment because the drug enters the bloodstream, travels through the body, and can kill cancer cells outside the pancreas.

Biological therapy tries to get the body to fight its own cancer. It uses materials made by the body or made in a laboratory to boost, direct, or rest the body's natural defenses against disease. Biological therapy is sometimes called biological response modifier (BRM) therapy or immunotherapy. It is being tested in clinical trials.

Patients may receive treatment that is considered standard based on its effectiveness in a number of patients in past studies, or may choose to go into a clinical trial. Most patients with cancer of the pancreas are not cured with standard therapy, and some standard treatments have undesirable side effects. Clinical trials are designed to find better ways to treat cancer patients and are based on the most up-to-date information. Clinical trials are taking place in most parts of the country for all stages of cancer of the pancreas. For more information, call the Cancer Information Service at 1-800-4-CANCER.

TREATMENT BY STAGE

STAGE I   Treatment may be one of the following:
                          1. Surgery to remove the head of the pan-
                             creas, part of the small intestine, and

some of the surrounding tissues (Whipple procedure).

2. Surgery to remove the entire pancreas and the organs around it (total pancreatectomy).
3. Surgery to remove the tail of the pancreas (distal pancreatectomy).
4. Surgery followed by chemotherapy and radiation therapy.
5. Clinical trials of radiation therapy given before, during, or after surgery.

STAGE II   Treatment may be one of the following:

1. Surgery or other treatments to reduce symptoms.
2. External-beam radiation therapy plus chemotherapy.
3. Clinical trials of radiation therapy plus drugs to make cancer cells more sensitive to radiation (radiosensitizers).
4. Clinical trials of radiation therapy given during surgery with internal radiation therapy.
5. Clinical trials of new types of radiation therapy.
6. Clinical trials of chemotherapy.
7. Clinical trials of surgery followed by external-beam radiation therapy and chemotherapy.

STAGE III   Treatment may be one of the following:

1. Surgery or other treatments to reduce symptoms.
2. External-beam radiation therapy and chemotherapy to reduce symptoms.
3. Clinical trials of surgery plus radiation therapy plus drugs to make cancer cells more sensitive to radiation (radiosensitizers).
4. Clinical trials of radiation therapy given during surgery, with or without removal of the cancer.

5. Clinical trials of new types of radiation therapy.

6. Clinical trials of chemotherapy.

STAGE IV   Treatment may be one of the following:

1. Surgery or other treatments to reduce symptoms.

2. Treatments for pain.

3. Clinical trials of chemotherapy or biological therapy.

RECURRENT   Treatment may be one of the following:

1. Chemotherapy.

2. Surgery to reduce symptoms.

3. External-beam radiation therapy to reduce symptoms.

4. Treatments for pain.

5. Clinical trials of chemotherapy or biological therapy.

To learn more about cancer of the pancreas, call the National Cancer Institute's Cancer Information Service at 1-800-4-CANCER. The Cancer Information Service can also send the following free booklets about cancer of the pancreas:

What You Need to Know About Cancer of the Pancreas
Research Report: Cancer of the Pancreas

The following chart summarizes the current facts about cancer of the pancreas.

CANCER OF THE PANCREAS

STATUS	28,100 new cases in the United States during 1990
	Accounts for approximately 3% of all cancers
INCIDENCE	Decreased 2% between 1973 and 1987
MORTALITY	Decreased approximately 5.6% between 1973 and 1987
	Lowest 5-year survival rate (3% for all stages) of any cancer
KNOWN CAUSE	Tobacco; certain industrial chemicals such as benzidine and beta-naphthylamine
LIFESTYLE CHANGES TO PREVENT THE CANCER	Stop smoking even low-tar cigarettes
	Increase consumption of fruits and leafy vegetables that contain beta-carotene
MEDICAL INTERVENTION	Encourage lifestyle changes above
	Explain importance of avoiding long-term exposure to industrial chemicals
RESEARCH FRONTIERS	Possible screening tests that use monoclonal antibodies to detect antigens on cancer cells

Chapter 18

Leukemia

LEUKEMIA IS A CANCER OF THE BLOOD CELLS. IT IS THE TENTH MOST common cancer in the United States. Nearly 28,000 new cases were diagnosed in 1990, accounting for about 3 percent of all cancers. Although most people consider leukemia to be a childhood disease, in fact the majority of those with the disease are adults and more than half of all leukemias occur in patients over sixty years of age. In the United States, leukemia occurs more often in whites than in blacks, and there is a somewhat higher incidence in males and people of Jewish descent than among other groups. It tends to occur in individuals who were exposed to ionizing radiation and certain chemicals and drugs, as well as in those with genetic abnormalities such as Down syndrome.

Leukemia is classified as acute (progressing rapidly) or chronic (progressing slowly). In *acute leukemia*, there is an abnormal growth of immature cells called blasts. In *chronic leukemia*, there are some blast cells but also an excessive number of mature blood cells. Leukemia is also classified according to the type of white blood cells that is abnormal in each form of the disease. Thus in lymphocytic leukemia the lymphocytes are abnormal, while in myelocytic (granulocytic) leukemia the myelocytes are abnormal.

Acute leukemias are subdivided into two categories: acute lymphocytic leukemia (ALL) and acute nonlymphocytic leukemia (ANLL). ANLL also includes other types of white cells, such as myelocytes (AML). About 75 percent of new acute leukemia cases each year are in adults over the age of sixty-five. Most adult leukemias are chronic, however, while 85 percent of childhood leukemia is acute. Chronic leukemias are also subdivided into two categories: chronic lymphocytic leukemia (CLL) and chronic myelocytic leukemia (CML). CLL is the most common leukemia and occurs mainly in individuals in their seventies. It is twice as common in men as in women.

In the past, untreated acute leukemias were rapidly fatal, while chronic leukemias progressed slowly. The prognosis for acute leukemia, especially in children, has greatly improved, and even the prognosis for chronic leukemias has improved somewhat. The mortality rate for all leukemias decreased 10 percent between 1973 and 1987. Because of the complexities and expense of administering proper care to the leukemic patient, anyone diagnosed with leukemia should be referred to a center that specializes in leukemia treatment.

Leukemia is a complex disease mainly because of the effects caused by the unregulated growth of lymphocytes. Lymphocytes are made by the bone marrow and by other organs of the lymph system. The bone marrow is the spongy tissue inside the large bones of the body. It makes red blood cells (which carry oxygen and other materials to all tissues of the body), white blood cells (which fight infection), and platelets (which make blood clot). Normally, the bone marrow makes cells called *blasts* that develop into several different types of blood cells, each with a specific function.

The lymph system is made up of thin tubes that branch, like blood cells, into all parts of the body. Lymph vessels carry lymph, a colorless, watery fluid that contains lymphocytes. Along the network of vessels are groups of small, bean-shaped organs called lymph nodes. Clusters of lymph nodes are found in the underarm, pelvis, neck, and abdomen. The spleen (an organ in the upper abdomen that makes lymphocytes and filters old blood cells from the blood), the thymus (a small organ beneath the sternum), and the tonsils (organs in the throat) are also part of the lymph system.

Lymphocytes fight infection by making substances called antibodies, which attack harmful bacteria in the body. In acute leukemia, the developing lymphocytes do not mature. These numerous immature lymphocytes make their way into the blood and the bone marrow. They also collect in the lymph tissues, making them swell. Lymphocytes may crowd out other blood cells in the blood and bone marrow. If the bone marrow cannot make enough red blood cells, the patient may have anemia. If the bone marrow cannot make enough platelets to make blood clot normally, the patient may bleed or bruise easily. The cancerous lymphocytes can also invade other organs, the spinal cord, and the brain.

Seven types of leukemia will be discussed in this chapter:

1. Adult acute lymphocytic leukemia (adult ALL)
2. Adult acute myeloid leukemia (adult AML)
3. Childhood acute lymphocytic leukemia (childhood ALL)
4. Childhood acute myeloid leukemia (childhood AML)
5. Chronic lymphocytic leukemia (CLL)
6. Chronic myelogenous leukemia (CML)
7. Hairy-cell leukemia (HCL)

The following list explains screening, diagnosis, and examinations for all leukemias.

Screening

No screening tests are currently available for leukemia, although routine physical examinations and blood tests may suggest the diagnosis. Dentists sometimes identify the disease.

Diagnosis

Leukemia is not usually difficult to diagnose, but a blood picture resembling leukemia may be present in some infections such as infectious mononucleosis, whooping cough, and tuberculosis.

Symptoms
Weakness, paleness
Fever and flulike symptoms
Bruising and prolonged bleeding
Enlarged lymph nodes, spleen, and liver
Pain in bones and joints
Frequent infections
Weight loss
Night sweats

Physical Examination   After eliciting a health history, the physician
will make a complete physical examination to detect fever, pallor,
bruises, bleeding from gums, bone or joint tenderness, and enlarged
lymph nodes, liver, or spleen.

Routine Laboratory Tests

Complete blood tests for the numbers of all cell types—red blood
cells, white blood cells, and platelets—and any abnormal or blast
cells

Blood chemistries, including coagulation factors

Urine analysis

Chest X rays, anterior and lateral views

Special Laboratory Tests

Bone marrow biopsy to detect proportions of various cell types and
any abnormal or blast cells

Spinal tap to detect various types of abnormal cells in spinal fluid

Various histochemical stain reactions (such as sudan black) to characterize further the blast cells (peroxidase, periodic acid-Schiff
[PAS], and various esterase stains)

Transfusion workup of patient to determine blood type

Determine B-cell and T-cell surface markers

Although not all of these tests are required for each patient, enough
of them must be performed to obtain a specific diagnosis. The patient's prognosis and future treatment depend on the specific cell type
of the leukemia and the patient's age and general health. Stages and
treatment of the seven types of leukemia to be considered are discussed in the separate sections that follow.

Adult Acute Lymphocytic Leukemia

Adult acute lymphocytic leukemia (also called acute lymphoblastic
leukemia or ALL) is a disease in which too many abnormal lymphocytes are found in the blood and bone marrow.

Like most cancers, acute adult lymphocytic leukemia is best treated
when it is found early. Unfortunately, it is often difficult to diagnose.
The early signs may be similar to those of the flu or other common
diseases. Anyone with a persistent fever, chronic weakness or tiredness, achy bones or joints, or swollen lymph nodes should see a
physician.

STAGES OF ADULT ACUTE LYMPHOCYTIC LEUKEMIA

There is no staging for adult acute lymphocytic leukemia. The choice of treatment depends on whether or not the patient has been treated.

UNTREATED	Untreated ALL means no specific anti-leukemic treatment has been given. There are too many white blood cells, including more than 5 percent blasts, in the blood and bone marrow, and there may be other signs and symptoms.
REMISSION	Treatment has been given, and the number of white blood cells and other blood cells in the blood and bone marrow has returned to normal. There are no signs or symptoms of leukemia.
RELAPSED/REFRACTORY	Relapsed disease means the leukemia has come back (recurred) after going into remission; refractory disease means the leukemia has failed to go into remission following treatment.

TREATMENT OF ADULT ACUTE LYMPHOCYTIC LEUKEMIA

There are treatments for all patients with adult ALL. The primary treatment is chemotherapy. Radiation therapy may be used in certain cases, and bone marrow transplantation is being studied in clinical trials.

Chemotherapy uses drugs to kill cancer cells. Chemotherapy may be taken by pill, or it may be put into the body by a needle in a vein or muscle. Chemotherapy is called a systemic treatment because the drug enters the bloodstream, travels through the body, and can kill cancer cells throughout the body. Chemotherapy may sometimes be put into the fluid that surrounds the brain through a needle in the brain or back (intrathecal chemotherapy).

Radiation therapy uses X rays or other high-energy rays to kill cancer cells and shrink tumors. Radiation for ALL usually comes from a machine outside the body (external-beam radiation therapy).

There are two phases of treatment for ALL. The first stage is called *induction therapy.* The purpose of induction therapy is to kill as many of the leukemia cells as possible and make the patient go into remission. Once in remission with no signs of leukemia, the patient receives a second phase of treatment, called *continuation therapy,* which tries to kill any remaining leukemia cells. Chemotherapy may continue for several years to keep the patient in remission.

If the leukemia cells have spread to the brain, the patient will receive radiation or chemotherapy to the brain. During induction and remission, the patient may also receive therapy to prevent leukemia cells from growing in the brain. This is called *central nervous system (CNS) prophylaxis.*

Bone marrow transplantation is a newer type of treatment that destroys all of the bone marrow in the body with high doses of chemotherapy with or without radiation therapy. Healthy marrow is then taken from another person (a donor) whose tissue is the same or almost the same as the patient's. The donor may be a twin (the best match), a sibling, or an unrelated person. The healthy marrow from the donor is given to the patient through a needle in the vein, to replace the marrow that was destroyed. A bone marrow transplant using marrow from a relative or an unrelated person is called an *allogeneic* bone marrow transplant. If it is from an identical twin, it is called a *syngeic* transplant.

A new type of bone marrow transplant, called *autologous* bone marrow transplant, is being studied in clinical trials. During this transplant, bone marrow is taken from the patient and treated with drugs to kill any cancer cells. The marrow is then frozen and the patient is given high-dose chemotherapy with or without radiation therapy to destroy all of the remaining marrow. The marrow that was taken out is then thawed and given to the patient through a needle in a vein to replace the marrow that was destroyed.

Treatment for adult lymphocytic leukemia depends on the patient's age and overall condition. The patient may receive treatment that is considered standard based on its effectiveness in a number of patients in past studies, or may choose to go into a clinical trial. Not all patients are cured with standard therapy, and some standard treatments may have undesirable side effects. Clinical trials are designed to find better ways to treat cancer patients and are based on the most up-to-date information. Clinical trials are taking place in most parts of the country for most stages of ALL. For more information, call the Cancer Information Service at 1-800-4-CANCER.

Treatment by Stage

UNTREATED

Treatment will probably be systemic chemotherapy. The patient may also receive intrathecal chemotherapy plus radiation therapy to the brain or high doses of systemic chemotherapy to treat or prevent leukemia in the brain. Clinical trials are testing new drugs.

REMISSION

Treatment may be one of the following:

1. Systemic chemotherapy. Intrathecal chemotherapy plus either radiation to the brain or high doses of systemic chemotherapy are also given to prevent leukemia cells from growing in the brain.
2. Clinical trials of bone marrow transplantation.
3. Clinical trials of new chemotherapy drugs.

RELAPSED

The patient may choose to take part in a clinical trial of new chemotherapy drugs or bone marrow transplantation.

To learn more about adult acute lymphocytic leukemia, call the National Cancer Institute's Cancer Information Service at 1-800-4-CANCER. The Cancer Information Service can also send the following free booklets:

Research Report: Leukemia
What You Need to Know About Adult Leukemia

Adult Acute Myeloid Leukemia

Adult acute myeloid leukemia (AML) is the most common form of acute leukemia in adults. In this disease, cancer cells are found in the blood and bone marrow. AML is also called acute nonlymphocytic leukemia or ANLL. It may be seen in patients at any age but primarily occurs between the ages of twenty and fifty-five.

Normally, the bone marrow makes cells called blasts that develop (mature) into several different types of blood cells that have specific jobs to do in the body. AML affects the blasts that are developing into white blood cells called granulocytes. In AML, the blasts do not mature and become too numerous. These immature blast cells are then found in the blood and the bone marrow.

The stages of adult acute myeloid leukemia are the same as those for adult acute lymphocytic leukemia. Its treatment is, in general, also the same as that for adult acute lymphocytic leukemia. Different chemotherapeutic agents may be used, however. Clinical trials are taking place in most parts of the country for most stages of adult AML. For more information, call the Cancer Information Service at 1-800-4-CANCER.

Childhood Acute Lymphocytic Leukemia

Childhood acute lymphocytic leukemia (also called acute lymphoblastic leukemia, or ALL) is a disease in which too many immature infection-fighting white blood cells, called lymphocytes, are found in the child's blood and bone marrow. ALL accounts for 85 percent of leukemia in children and is the most common kind of childhood cancer. It occurs mostly between the ages of two and eight, more often in boys than in girls. It is also the most treatable of all leukemias.

The stages of childhood acute lymphocytic leukemia are the same as those for acute adult lymphocytic leukemia.

TREATMENT OF CHILDHOOD ACUTE LYMPHOCYTIC LEUKEMIA

There are three phases of treatment for ALL. The first phase is called *induction therapy*. The purpose of induction therapy is to kill as many of the leukemia cells as possible and to make the child go into remission. Once the child goes into remission and there are no signs of leukemia, a second phase of treatment is given, called *consolidation therapy*, which tries to kill any remaining leukemia cells. A third phase of treatment, called *maintenance therapy*, may be given for up to several years to keep the child in remission.

If the leukemia cells have spread to the brain, the child will receive chemotherapy with radiation therapy to the brain. During induction and maintenance, the child may also receive therapy to prevent leukemia cells from growing in the brain. This type of therapy is called *central nervous system (CNS) prophylaxis.*

Bone marrow transplantation is a newer type of treatment and is described in the section on adult acute ALL.

Treatment by Stage   Treatment for childhood ALL depends on the prognostic group the child is assigned to, based on the child's age, white cell count, and other factors.

UNTREATED	The child's treatment will probably be systemic chemotherapy. The child will also receive some type of therapy to treat or prevent leukemia in the brain. This therapy may be intrathecal chemotherapy with or without radiation therapy to the brain, or high doses of systemic chemotherapy with intrathecal chemotherapy. Clinical trials are testing new drugs and new ways of treatment and preventing leukemia in the brain.
REMISSION	The child's treatment will probably be systemic chemotherapy. Intrathecal and/or high doses of systemic chemotherapy is given to prevent leukemia cells from growing in the brain.
RELAPSED	The child's treatment depends on the type of treatment the child received before, how soon the cancer came back following treatment, and whether the leukemia cells are found outside the bone marrow. The child's treatment will probably be systemic chemotherapy. The parents may want to consider a clinical trial of new chemotherapy drugs or bone marrow transplantation for the child.

If clinical trials show that the new treatment is better than the one being used, the new treatment may become standard. Children who are treated in clinical trials have the advantage of getting the best therapy available. In the United States, about two-thirds of children with cancer are treated in a clinical trial at some point in their illness.

In the United States, there are two major groups (called cooperative groups) that organize clinical trials for childhood cancers: the Children's Cancer Study Group (CCSG) and the Pediatric Oncology Group (POG). Doctors who belong to these groups or who take part in other clinical trials are listed in PDQ.

Parents can use PDQ to learn more about current treatments for their children's cancer. Parents should take this material from PDQ with them when they see the child's physician and talk to the physician about which treatment would be best.

To learn more about childhood acute lymphocytic leukemia, call the National Cancer Institute's Cancer Information Service at 1-800-4-CANCER. The Cancer Information Service can also send free booklets:

Research Report: Leukemia
Research Report: Bone Marrow Transplantation

The following booklets on childhood cancer may also be helpful:

Young People with Cancer: A Handbook for Parents
Talking with Your Child About Cancer
Diet and Nutrition: A Resource for Parents of Children with Cancer
Hospital Days, Treatment Ways (Coloring Book)
Help Yourself: Tips for Teenagers with Cancer

There are many other places where parents can get material about cancer treatment and services. The American Cancer Society and the Leukemia Society of America have information and services for leukemia patients. Candlelighters Childhood Cancer Foundation (1-800-366-2223) has free services and publications including newsletters, bibliographies, and information for parents and brothers and sisters of children with cancer. It can also refer parents to a parent peer support group in the United States or abroad. Local offices for these organizations are listed in the white pages of the telephone book.

Childhood Acute Myeloid Leukemia

Childhood acute myeloid leukemia (AML) is a disease in which cancer cells are found in the child's blood and bone marrow. AML is also called acute nonlymphocytic leukemia, or ANLL. It is less common than childhood acute lymphocytic leukemia.

Normally, the bone marrow makes cells called blasts that develop into several different types of blood cells that have specific functions in the body. AML affects the blasts that are developing into white blood cells called granulocytes, which fight infection. The blasts do not mature. These numerous immature blast cells then make their way into the blood and the bone marrow.

Acute myeloid leukemia progresses quickly. A treatable and sometimes curable cancer, it can occur in children of any age. The stages of childhood acute myeloid leukemia are the same as those for adult acute lymphocytic leukemia. Its primary treatment is chemotherapy, sometimes followed by bone marrow transplantation. Radiation therapy may be used in certain cases.

There are two phases of treatment for AML. The first phase is called *induction therapy.* The purpose of induction therapy is to kill as many of the leukemia cells as possible and make the child go into remission. Once the child goes into remission and there are no signs of leukemia, a second phase of treatment is given, called *postremission therapy,* which tries to kill any remaining leukemia cells. Chemotherapy may be given for several years to keep the child in remission.

If the leukemia cells have spread to the brain, the child will receive radiation therapy to the brain, or intrathecal chemotherapy. During induction and remission, the child may also receive therapy to prevent leukemia cells from growing in the brain. This is called *central nervous system (CNS) prophylaxis.*

Bone marrow transplantation is a newer type of treatment for childhood AML. It was described earlier as a treatment for acute adult ALL.

TREATMENT BY STAGE

UNTREATED	The child's treatment will probably be systemic chemotherapy—intrathecal chemotherapy with or without radiation therapy to the brain.
REMISSION	The child's treatment may be one of the following:
	Bone marrow transplantation (autologous or allogenic)

Systemic chemotherapy
Clinical trials are comparing these two
treatments to find out whether one is better than the other.

RELAPSED   Treatment depends on the type of treatment the child received before. The parent
may want to have the child take part in a
clinical trial of new chemotherapy drugs or
bone marrow transplantation. Clinical trials organized by the Children's Cancer
Study Group and the Pediatric Oncology
Group were described earlier.

To learn more about childhood acute myeloid leukemia, call the
National Cancer Institute's Cancer Information Service at 1-800-4-
CANCER. See the section on childhood acute lymphocytic leukemia
for information on free booklets available on childhood leukemia.
Other materials are available from the American Cancer Society, the
Leukemia Society of America, and the Candlelighters Childhood Can-
cer Foundation.

Chronic Lymphocytic Leukemia

Chronic lymphocytic leukemia (CLL) is the most common leukemia.
It is a disease in which large numbers of infection-fighting white blood
cells called lymphocytes are found in the body.

Lymphocytes fight infection by making substances called antibodies, which attack viruses, bacteria, and other harmful things in the
body. In CLL, the developing lymphocytes do not mature correctly,
and too many are made. The lymphocytes may look normal, but they
cannot fight infection as well as they should. These immature lymphocytes make their way into the blood and the bone marrow. They
also collect in the lymph tissues and make them swell. Lymphocytes
may crowd out other blood cells in the blood and bone marrow. If the
bone marrow cannot make enough red blood cells to carry oxygen, the
patient may have anemia. If the bone marrow cannot make enough
platelets to make the blood clot normally, the patient may bleed or
bruise easily.

Chronic lymphocytic leukemia progresses slowly and usually occurs in people sixty years of age or older. It is twice as common in men

than in women. In the first stages of the disease, there are often no symptoms. As time goes on, more and more lymphocytes are made and symptoms begin to appear. Anyone whose lymph nodes swell, whose spleen or liver becomes larger than normal, who feels tired all the time, or who bleeds easily should see a physician. Loss of appetite and weight loss should also send one to a physician.

STAGES OF CHRONIC LYMPHOCYTIC LEUKEMIA

When chronic lymphocytic leukemia has been diagnosed, more tests may be done to find out whether leukemia cells have spread to other parts of the body. This is called staging. The physician needs to know the stage of the disease in order to plan treatment. The stages of chronic lymphocytic leukemia are named as follows:

STAGE O
There are too many lymphocytes in the blood, but there are usually no other symptoms of leukemia. Lymph nodes and the spleen and liver are not swollen, and the number of red blood cells and platelets is normal.

STAGE I
There are too many lymphocytes in the blood, and lymph nodes are swollen. The spleen and liver are not swollen, and the number of blood cells and platelets is normal.

STAGE II
There are too many lymphocytes in the blood, and lymph nodes and the liver and spleen are swollen.

STAGE III
There are too many lymphocytes in the blood, and there are too few red blood cells (anemia). Lymph nodes and the liver or spleen may be swollen.

STAGE IV
There are too many lymphocytes in the blood and too few platelets, which makes it hard for the blood to clot. The lymph nodes, liver, or spleen may be swollen, and there may be too few red blood cells (anemia).

REFRACTORY
The leukemia does not respond to treatment.

TREATMENT OF CHRONIC LYMPHOCYTIC LEUKEMIA

Three kinds of treatment are generally used: chemotherapy, radiation therapy, and treatment for complications of the leukemia, such as infection. The use of biological therapy (using the body's immune system to fight cancer) is being tested in clinical trials. Surgery may be used in certain cases. If the spleen is swollen, for example, the surgeon may take out the spleen in an operation called a *splenectomy*, but this is done only in rare cases. A person can function normally without a spleen, but runs an increased risk of certain infections.

Biological therapy tries to get the patient's own body to fight cancer. It uses materials made by the body or made in a laboratory to boost, direct, or restore the body's natural defenses against disease. Biological therapy is sometimes called biological response modifier (BRM) therapy or immunotherapy.

Because infections often occur in patients with CLL, a special substance called immunoglobulin, which contains antibodies, may be given to prevent infections. Sometimes a special machine is used to filter the blood to take out extra lymphocytes. This is called *leukopheresis*.

Treatment by Stage

STAGE O	The patient usually does not need treatment. The physician will follow the patient closely so that treatment can begin if the leukemia gets worse.
STAGE I	Treatment may be one of the following: 1. If there are no symptoms, no treatment is needed. The physician will follow the patient closely so that treatment can begin if the leukemia gets worse. 2. External-beam radiation therapy to swollen lymph nodes. 3. Chemotherapy.
STAGE II	Treatment may be one of the following: 1. Chemotherapy. 2. Clinical trials of biological therapy. 3. Clinical trials of external radiation therapy to the spleen.
STAGE III	Treatment may be one of the following:

1. Chemotherapy. Clinical trials are testing new drugs and combinations of drugs.
2. Splenectomy.
3. Clinical trials of external-beam radiation therapy to the whole body (whole body radiation).
4. Clinical trials of biological therapy.
5. Clinical trials of leukopheresis.
6. Clinical trials of external-beam radiation therapy to the spleen.

STAGE IV   Treatment may be one of the following:
1. Chemotherapy. Clinical trials are testing new drugs and combinations of drugs.
2. Splenectomy.
3. Clinical trials of external-beam radiation therapy to the whole body (whole body radiation).
4. Clinical trials of biological therapy.
5. Clinical trials of external-beam radiation therapy to the spleen.

REFRACTORY   Treatment depends on many factors. The patient may wish to consider entering a clinical trial of new chemotherapy drugs.

To learn more about chronic lymphocytic leukemia, call the National Cancer Institute's Cancer Information Service at 1-800-4-CANCER. The Cancer Information Service can also send the following free booklets about leukemia:

Research Report: Leukemia
What You Need to Know About Adult Leukemia

Chronic Myelogenous Leukemia

Chronic myelogenous leukemia (also called CML or chronic granulocytic leukemia) is a disease in which too many white blood cells are made in the bone marrow.

CML affects the blasts that are developing into white blood cells called granulocytes. The blasts do not mature and become too numerous. These immature blast cells make their way into the blood and the bone marrow. In most people with CML, the genetic material (chromosomes) in the leukemia cells has a feature that is not normal, called a Philadelphia chromosome. This chromosome usually doesn't go away, even after treatment.

Chronic myelogenous leukemia progresses slowly and usually occurs in people who are middle-aged or older, although it can occur in children. It occurs slightly more in males than in females. In the first stages of CML, most people don't have any symptoms of cancers. They should see a physician if they notice any of the following: tiredness that won't go away, a feeling of having no energy, fever, loss of appetite, or night sweats. The spleen may be swollen.

STAGES OF CHRONIC MYELOGENOUS LEUKEMIA

When chronic myelogenous leukemia has been diagnosed, more tests may be done to find out whether leukemia cells have spread to other parts of the body, such as the brain. This is called staging. The physician needs to know the stages of the disease in order to plan treatment. The stages of chronic myelogenous leukemia are named as follows:

CHRONIC PHASE — There are no more than 5 percent blast cells in the blood and bone marrow, and there may be no symptoms of leukemia. This phase may last from several months to several years.

ACCELERATED PHASE — There are more blast cells (5 percent to 30 percent) and fewer normal cells in the blood and bone marrow.

BLASTIC PHASE — Sometimes called "blast crisis." More than 30 percent of the cells in the blood or bone marrow are blast cells. Sometimes blast cells will form tumors outside the bone marrow, such as in the bone or lymph nodes.

MENINGEAL — Leukemia cells are found in the fluid that surrounds the brain and/or spinal cord. Meningeal CML can occur during the accelerated phase or the blastic phase.

REFRACTORY   Leukemia cells do not decrease, even after
                              treatment.

TREATMENT OF CHRONIC MYELOGENOUS LEUKEMIA

The kinds of treatment are the same as for acute childhood lymphocytic leukemia.

Treatment by Stage

CHRONIC PHASE   Treatment may be one of the following:
                              1. No treatment if blood counts are nearly
                                 normal. The physician will follow the
                                 patient closely so that treatment can
                                 begin if the disease is progressing.
                              2. Chemotherapy to lower the number of
                                 white blood cells.
                              3. Splenectomy.
                              4. Bone marrow transplantation.
                              5. Clinical trials of biological therapy.

ACCELERATED PHASE   Treatment may be one of the following:
                              1. Chemotherapy to lower the number of
                                 white blood cells.
                              2. Transfusions of blood or blood products
                                 to relieve symptoms.
                              3. Clinical trials of bone marrow transplan-
                                 tation.

BLASTIC PHASE   Treatment may be one of the following:
                              1. Chemotherapy. Clinical trials are test-
                                 ing new chemotherapy drugs and new
                                 combinations of drugs.
                              2. Radiation therapy to relieve symptoms
                                 caused by tumors formed in the bone.
                              3. Clinical trials of bone marrow transplan-
                                 tation.

MENINGEAL   Treatment may be one of the following:
                              1. Intrathecal chemotherapy.
                              2. Radiation therapy to the brain.

REFRACTORY   Treatment depends on many factors. The
                        patient may wish to consider entering a
                        clinical trial.

To learn more about chronic myelogenous leukemia, call the National Cancer Institute's Cancer Information Service at 1-800-4-CANCER.

Hairy-Cell Leukemia

Hairy-cell leukemia (HCL) is a disease in which malignant cells are found in the blood and bone marrow. The disease is so named because the cancer cells look "hairy" when examined under a microscope. Usually found in elderly patients, hairy-cell leukemia is an uncommon B-cell neoplasm characterized by low numbers of all types of blood cells—red, white, and platelets—and an enlarged spleen without enlarged lymph nodes. Because HCL causes lower numbers of white blood cells, patients are prone to develop many types of infection. Before the discovery of effective treatment, some patients had prolonged survival after splenectomy.

There is no staging system for hairy-cell leukemia. Patients are categorized based on whether or not they have been treated.

UNTREATED   No treatment has been given for the leuke-
                        mia. Treatment may have been given
                        for infections or other side effects of the
                        leukemia.
PROGRESSIVE,   Surgery has been done to remove the spleen
POST-SPLENECTOMY   (splenectomy) but the leukemia is getting
                        worse.
REFRACTORY   The leukemia has been treated but no lon-
                        ger responds to the treatment.

TREATMENT OF HAIRY-CELL LEUKEMIA

Some patients with hairy-cell leukemia have few symptoms and may not need treatment right away. There are treatments for all patients with hairy-cell leukemia that is causing symptoms. Three kinds of treatment are generally used: surgery, chemotherapy, and biological therapy. Bone marrow transplants are being tested in clinical trials.

Treatment by Category

UNTREATED

Treatment may be one of the following:
1. If there are no symptoms, no treatment may be needed. The physician will follow the patient closely so that treatment can begin if the leukemia gets worse.
2. Splenectomy.
3. Biological therapy using interferon.
4. Clinical trials of chemotherapy.
5. Clinical trials comparing chemotherapy and biological therapy.

PROGRESSIVE, POST-SPLENECTOMY

Treatment may be one of the following:
1. Biological therapy.
2. Chemotherapy. Clinical trials are testing new chemotherapy drugs.
3. Clinical trials comparing biological therapy and chemotherapy.
4. Clinical trials of bone marrow transplantation.
5. Leukopheresis to lower the number of white blood cells.

REFRACTORY

Patients who do not respond to biological therapy may receive chemotherapy. They may also elect to take part in a clinical trial of new chemotherapy drugs.

To learn more about hairy-cell leukemia, call the National Cancer Institute's Cancer Information Service at 1-800-4-CANCER.

The following chart summarizes the current facts about leukemias.

LEUKEMIA

STATUS	27,800 new cases in the United States during 1990
	Accounts for approximately 3% of all cancers
INCIDENCE	Decreased 5.6% between 1973 and 1987
MORTALITY	Decreased 10% between 1973 and 1987
	30% to 35% of adults with acute leukemia are cured
	5-year survival rate for children with all types of leukemia was 67% from 1981 to 1987
KNOWN CAUSES	X rays and ionizing radiation from atomic bomb
	16% of all leukemias in the United States may be caused by diagnostic X rays. For instance, diagnostic X rays to the trunk of the body cause chronic myelogenous leukemia and possibly acute myelogenous leukemia.
	HTLV-I viruses cause adult T-cell leukemia, and HTLV-II may cause hairy-cell leukemia.
	Benzene and certain anticancer drugs, as well as certain diseases with chromosome aberrations, such as Down syndrome, Bloom's syndrome, and Fanconi's anemia, predispose to leukemia.
LIFESTYLE CHANGES TO PREVENT LEUKEMIA	Avoid exposure to chemicals such as benzene.
MEDICAL INTERVENTION	Advise against exposure to chemicals such as benzene.
	Monitor the use of diagnostic and therapeutic X rays.
	Monitor long-term survivors who received certain chemotherapeutic drugs for leukemia.
	Observe patients with Down syndrome and other genetic diseases for leukemia.
	Use drugs such as chloramphenicol only when specifically indicated.

Research studies have identified a number of characteristics of the acute leukemia patient at the time of initial diagnosis that are important for prognosis and for type of treatment. These factors include age, high white blood cell count, the presence of meningeal leukemia or infection, B-cell markers on lymphocytes, and presence of Philadelphia chromosome.

Various chromosomal changes found in ANNL cells may impair response to chemotherapy and influence the prognosis.

In acute lymphocytic leukemia, the detection of fusion of two oncogenes (bcr and abl) yields an accurate diagnosis, distinguishes it from other leukemias, and aids in selection of optimal treatment.

In chronic myelogenous leukemia, the detection of fusion of two oncogenes (bcr and abl) also aids in diagnosis.

The use of a new technique called polymerase chain reaction can be used to detect residual leukemia cells in a treated patient. Such detection is an important guide to appropriate treatment.

The origins of certain leukemias have been associated with translocation of protooncogenes to regions of active immunoglobulin genes or T-cell receptor genes. In chronic lymphocytic leukemia the bcl protooncogenes on chromosome 11, after translocation to chromosome 14, are activated by the immunoglobulin gene. Similarly in T-cell leukemia the *myc* protooncogene on chromosome 8 is activated after translocation to chromosome 14, by the T-cell receptor gene.

Studies are under way to evaluate the MLL gene as a marker in leukemic cells of infants with acute lymphoblastic leukemia; if present, treatment should be more aggressive.

Treatment of acute promyelocytic leukemia with retinoic acid derivations is under way.

Epilogue

How We Wage the War on Cancer

M ANY PEOPLE SHARE THE PESSIMISTIC VIEWS THAT CANCER IS INCREAS-ing in incidence and that current treatments are often ineffective. But new information clearly indicates that many of the most common cancers can be prevented by lifestyle changes, and many types of medical intervention and treatment are indeed successful. Despite this hopeful turn of events, cancer is now the leading cause of death in women and, if current trends continue, will be the leading cause of death in both men and women in the United States, and perhaps other industrialized countries, by the end of the century.

This fact is not the result of continuing increases in cancer mortality but, rather, of the spectacular and consistent decline in deaths due to heart disease, which has been the major cause of death for the last forty years. In fact, the overall death rate from cancer has remained quite stable, while the death rate from heart disease has decreased by 45 percent (Henderson 1991)—thus the proportion of deaths attributable to cancer has become larger.

The huge decrease in heart disease mortality can serve as a model for our approach to cancer. The success story of heart disease was made possible by a combination of lifestyle changes, preventive measures, and improved treatments. People started smoking less, lowering their intake of fat and cholesterol, and becoming aware of the dangers of the "silent killer," high blood pressure, and willing to take new drugs on a daily basis to lower blood pressure. A vast array of ingenious surgical and medical treatments became available to treat the clinical manifestations of heart disease.

Although, as just mentioned, there has been little change in overall cancer mortality during the last forty years, major changes have taken place in the incidence and mortality of certain individual cancers, as the accompanying chart shows. Between 1973 and 1987, greater than 15 percent increases in incidence and mortality have occurred in lung cancer, melanoma, multiple myeloma, and non-Hodgkin's lymphomas. The history of lung cancer is especially enlightening. It was only a rare cancer at the turn of the century. The upsurge in cigarette smoking from 1900 until the 1960s made it the leading cause of cancer death. Now lung cancer mortality in men has leveled off as fewer men smoke, but in 1986 lung cancer surpassed breast cancer as the leading cause of death in women, and death rates among women are predicted to increase for another ten years. Given this projected increase in deaths from lung cancer, cancer will become the leading cause of death by the year 2000, surpassing that from all other diseases.

CHANGES IN INCIDENCE AND MORTALITY OF VARIOUS CANCER SITES, 1973–1987

INCREASE IN INCIDENCE AND MORTALITY	Lung, melanoma, multiple myeloma, non-Hodgkin's lymphomas
INCREASE IN INCIDENCE, BUT SMALL CHANGES IN MORTALITY	Breast, prostate, kidney, brain, and other nervous-tissue cancers
INCREASING OR STABLE INCIDENCE, BUT DECREASING MORTALITY	Rectum, bladder, testes, thyroid, oral cavity, lip, and pharynx
STABLE INCIDENCE AND MORTALITY	Colon, ovary, pancreas, liver, esophagus, larynx, leukemia (and all other sites)
DECREASE IN BOTH INCIDENCE AND MORTALITY	Hodgkin's disease, stomach, cervix, uterus

SOURCE: Adapted from table in B. E. Henderson, R. K. Ross, and M. C. Pike, "Toward the Primary Prevention of Cancer," *Science* 254 (1991).

On the positive side, if a smoker quits, even after a heavy, long-term habit, the cancer risk will be greatly reduced. Low-tar cigarettes are associated with lower cancer risks than high-tar cigarettes, but smokers of low-tar cigarettes still have a much higher cancer risk than nonsmokers. Evidence is accumulating that passive smoking is also associated with a modestly increased risk of lung cancer. The overall contribution of passive smoking—in which nonsmokers are exposed to sidestream smoke from burning tobacco and mainstream smoke exhaled by smokers—is small, however. Smoking-prevention programs are increasingly successful. But because of the long-lasting effects of cigarette smoking and the continued smoking by a sizable minority of the population, lung cancer from this one factor will continue to be a major health problem for decades to come.

As noted in the chart, melanoma, multiple myeloma, and non-Hodgkin's lymphomas have also shown increases in incidence and mortality. The melanoma increases are caused mainly by increased exposure to sunlight, attributable to recreational habits and clothing design. For the other two cancers, the increases are unexplained but most likely are due to better diagnostic techniques that can distinguish these cancers.

Despite the increases in incidence in breast, prostate, kidney, and brain cancers, the mortality for these cancers decreased between 1973 and 1987. This is probably due to earlier detection and more effective treatment of these potentially fatal cancers. For instance, much of the increase in breast cancer incidence is due to the increased use of mammography because screening can detect small local lesions that are amenable to effective treatment. Similarly, early detection of prostate cancer during physical examinations and by other screening procedures may explain its increase in incidence. Effective treatment of local disease can explain the reduced mortality. The increase in kidney cancer is thought to be another consequence of cigarette smoking. The increase in brain tumors may be due to two factors. First, in the past dental X-ray equipment yielded much higher exposures than is experienced with the modern X-ray machine. Second, CT scans can diagnose small, "silent" brain tumors.

As for the third group on the chart, the large decrease in mortality from testicular cancer despite an even larger increase in incidence is an excellent example of the results of modern treatment, including chemotherapy. More effective treatments have also resulted in the decreases in mortality from rectal, bladder, thyroid, oral cavity, lip, and pharynx cancers.

Other types of cancers have declined in both incidence and mortality. The biggest success story is Hodgkin's disease, for which the decline in mortality is three times greater than the decline in incidence. The use of radiation therapy combined with chemotherapy has produced many permanent cures of this previously fatal disease. The decrease in stomach cancer has been observed for years and is believed to be related to changes in methods of food preservation and diet. Similarly, the long-standing decrease in cervical cancer mortality is related to early detection and treatment of premalignant or localized cervical lesions.

A dramatic increase in the incidence of uterine cancer in the early 1970s was attributed mainly to an increase in the administration of large doses of estrogen to postmenopausal women. Since then, a reduced dose of estrogen, along with progesterone, has been prescribed for older women and, among younger women, there has been an increased use of oral contraceptives (consisting of estrogens and progesterone). A decrease in the incidence and mortality rates of uterine cancer followed.

Only small changes in mortality and incidence have been observed in cancers of the colon, ovary, pancreas, and larynx and in leukemia. Some increase in the incidence of esophageal and liver cancer is thought to be caused by the combined effects of tobacco and alcohol. We would expect the incidence and mortality rates of various cancers to be constantly changing as new information about causes, prevention, and medical intervention is slowly tipping the scale toward control of the disease.

As has been made clear earlier in the book, cancer incidence and mortality rise sharply with age. For example, the death rate from cancer of the large intestine increases more than one thousand times between the ages of thirty and eighty. For most cancers, the interval between initial exposure to carcinogen and development of cancer may be decades rather than months or years. The current concept of carcinogenesis as a multistep process requiring separate mutations for the activation of protooncogenes to oncogenes and the loss or inactivation of a tumor-suppressor gene fits this correlation.

These mutations might occur spontaneously, which accounts for some 20 percent of cancers, or might be induced by environmental carcinogens, accounting for the remaining 80 percent. In the cancers that affect children and young adults, fewer alterations of protooncogenes and tumor-suppressor genes are required for the cancer to appear. Infants and young children who develop the six embryonal cancers (retinoblastoma, osteosarcoma, Wilms' tumor, rhabdomyosarcoma, hepatoblastoma, and neuroblastoma) have inherited only one functional copy of the usual pair of tumor-suppressor genes. When the second copy is altered (either spontaneously, during cell division, or by exposure to an X ray or chemical) early in life, the cancer develops. Similarly, young women who develop early-onset breast cancer may have inherited an inactive copy of the p53 tumor-suppressor gene, one of the steps in the progression toward cancer.

Because the mutation can occur at any time in the life of the cell or its ancestors, the probability of a mutation in a particular gene will increase with increasing age. Some historical examples will bear this out. Bladder cancer developed after an interval of many years in almost all workers heavily exposed to 2-naphthylamine around 1850. Leukemia reached its peak incidence seven years after individuals were exposed to the radiation caused by the explosion of atomic bombs in 1945. Other forms of cancer, such as breast cancer, increased in incidence ten to twenty years after women's exposure to radiation from the bombs. A delayed response related to hormone therapy was seen in women given diethylstilbestrol during pregnancy. Their daughters developed carcinoma of the vagina as teenagers. Lung cancer in older people is related to the duration and intensity of exposure to cigarette smoke. It is theorized that varying numbers of steps might be involved in different forms of cancer; the more steps, the longer the cancer will take to develop.

New Clinical Measures

EARLIER DIAGNOSIS

With current molecular diagnostic techniques, it is possible to test an individual's DNA and determine the status of some oncogenes and tumor-suppressor genes, which can indicate a predisposition to certain cancers. This ability to detect changes in these genes means early diagnoses and intervention.

A good example of this ability is hereditary retinoblastoma. In families known to have this tumor, a sample of fetal DNA can be tested to determine whether it is normal or has alterations in the Rb genes that would render the baby susceptible to the tumor. The baby could be observed carefully and treated immediately if a tumor appeared. Several such newborn babies whose small tumors were treated at about a month of age were cured (personal communication, A. Linn Murphree, M.D.).

Current tests are also useful in determining its progress once cancer has occurred, thus helping the physician design the most appropriate treatment. Children with neuroblastomas exhibiting amplified c-N-*myc* oncogene, for example, have a poor outlook for survival and must receive all available forms of treatment. Some molecular diagnostic techniques are already being applied to detect cancer in early states. Urine from patients with bladder cancer may contain cells with a defective p53 gene. Colon cells shed into the feces are being tested for defects in protooncogenes and tumor-suppressor genes. Such efforts may prove more useful in diagnosing certain cancers than standard methods, allowing for earlier, often more successful treatment.

Another new molecular genetic technique will be of help in testing patients with certain types of cancer, such as leukemia, for residual disease after they have received therapy. Called the polymerase chain reaction, this technique can amplify specific segments of cellular DNA. Once the DNA alteration in a patient's cancer cells is known, the exquisitely sensitive test can be applied to samples of cells after treatment, detecting any cancer cells that survived. For instance, in certain lymphomas an alteration in the location of the *bcl* oncogene can be discovered in 1 among 100,000 cells. Additional treatment could then be used to eradicate the rare residual lymphoma cell and prevent recurrence.

NEW TREATMENTS

How can the new information about retroviruses and the two sets of cancer genes be used to treat cancer? First, the extensive studies under way to treat patients with AIDS should have a direct bearing on the treatment of leukemia caused by HTLV-I and HTLV-II retroviruses, even though these viruses are only distantly related to HIV, the virus that causes AIDS. Antiviral agents such as AZT and ddI, and other drugs developed for AIDS, are likely to be useful in treating HTLV-induced leukemia.

The therapeutic strategy for treating the vast majority of cancers not caused by these retroviruses can be devised from determining the roles of oncogenes and tumor-suppressor genes and attacking them. The slow, multistep progression of these genetic events, if pinpointed, suggests that early intervention may be possible at various steps in the process. Understanding the pathways by which protooncogene products function may also be of help in devising new methods of cancer therapy. Compounds that inactivate the products of the genes or compete with them for their cellular receptors are examples of treatment strategies already planned to be tested.

Other strategies can be tested for tumor-suppressor genes. Laboratory studies have already demonstrated that Wilms' tumor cells grown *in vitro* can be changed into normal cells by the insertion of the tumor-suppressor gene on chromosome 11. Similar results were obtained when the Rb gene was inserted into cultured retinoblastomas or osteosarcoma cells. From these encouraging results, it is hoped that the Rb gene experimentally incorporated into a retrovirus can be inserted into the patient's retinoblastoma cells by infecting the tumor cells with the modified retrovirus. The infected cells would be converted into normal cells by the function of the product of the inserted Rb gene. Similar studies of other tumor-suppressor genes incorporated into herpes viruses are under way to determine whether brain tumor cells infected by the viruses can be converted into normal cells.

Recently, Bert Vogelstein and colleagues at Johns Hopkins University inserted a normal p53 gene into cultured human colon cells and reduced their proliferation. Such studies must be evaluated in light of the ethical constraints associated with genetic engineering techniques applied to humans and the obvious technical problem of inserting a healthy gene into all the cells in a tumor.

A final therapeutic strategy related to tumor-suppressor genes is to isolate their protein products and administer them as drugs to appropriate cancer patients. Thus, the Rb gene product (the purified 105 K protein) could be injected into tumors of patients in an effort to convert the tumor cells into normal cells.

Besides these types of gene therapy, it may be possible to develop drugs that will mimic the actions of tumor-suppressor genes such as Rb or p53. This is an important concept because these genes play a role in many types of cancer. Thus a single drug that stimulates cells to produce additional quantities of the p53 gene product could have a broad spectrum of usefulness.

A variety of biological therapies, or biological response modifiers, were studied during the 1980s. These drugs are laboratory-manufactured copies of substances found naturally in the body. Some have proven useful; for instance, almost one-third of melanoma patients respond successfully to the immunological therapies interleukin-2 and the lymphokine-activated killer cells (LAK). It is not known why the other two-thirds do not respond. While these agents were at first thought to be the "magic bullets" of cancer therapy, the expectations surrounding them have not been realized. They are now being used only selectively, especially to "mop up" after surgery, radiation, or chemotherapy.

One new agent, called granulocyte-colony stimulating factor (G-CSF), is used in cancer therapy after bone marrow transplantation, to stimulate regrowth of bone marrow and prevent infection.

In contrast to the disappointments about biological therapy, one new drug, taxol, has been discovered that may prove to be an important chemotherapeutic agent. Research on taxol as a chemotherapeutic agent began in the late 1970s, and the drug is only now becoming available in clinical trials. It has been found to be successful in treating ovarian and breast cancer and may be useful in lung and other cancers. In a recent study of forty-eight women with advanced ovarian cancer, sixteen showed a regression of the tumor and one woman's cancer disappeared (Greenspan 1991). A Food and Drug Administration panel has recently recommended that taxol be approved for the treatment of ovarian cancer (*New York Times*, November 17, 1992).

Taxol is made from the bark of the Pacific yew, found in forests in the northwest United States and British Columbia. The drug is painstaking to manufacture. The bark of about 38,000 trees is required to prepare 55 pounds of taxol, enough to treat 1,200 patients. Chemists have, of course, been attempting to synthesize taxol in the laboratory. They have not been able to replicate the entire taxol structure but have synthesized one segment, or "tail," of it. The other main segment, or body, has been discovered in native form, in the easily obtainable leaves of yew trees. If the native body and the synthetic tail can be joined and the resultant taxol structure proves to have anticancer activity, an important step will have been taken to provide more of this important new drug.

In addition to these new therapeutic strategies, other advances are being made in the combined use of bone marrow transplantation and chemotherapy, radiation therapy, and surgical therapy. These advances have resulted in increased cure rates for certain cancers, such as those of the breast and lung (see chart).

ADVANCES IN TREATMENT

Polychemotherapy

DEFINITION   Patient receives a combination of drugs to kill cancer cells by different mechanisms and to prevent the severe problem of cells becoming resistant to one drug.

EXAMPLE   Polychemotherapy of breast cancer has resulted in 10-year disease-free cures in 25%
to 30% of patients.

*High-Dose Chemotherapy Combined with
Bone Marrow Transplantation*

DEFINITION   Patient receives doses of chemotherapy
tenfold higher than normally given, plus
radiation. Thereafter, patient receives normal bone marrow from a donor, or the bone
marrow previously collected and stored
from the patient. The transplanted bone
marrow cells repopulate the bone marrow
with new red blood cells, white blood cells,
and platelets.

EXAMPLE   The treatment was first used for leukemia
and lymphoma patients. It is now used on
patients with neuroblastomas and advanced breast and testicular cancers.

Adjuvant Therapy

DEFINITION   Patient receives chemotherapy and/or radiation therapy before surgery in order to re-
duce the size of an otherwise inoperable
tumor. Such adjuvant therapy can also be
used after surgery to kill remaining cancer
cells.

EXAMPLE   Adjuvant therapy has increased lung cancer survival rates from 8% in 1980 to 15%.
It is widely used for many patients with
breast and testicular cancer and sarcomas.
It is sometimes used for colon and bladder
cancers.

Causes of Cancer Revisited

Epidemiological evidence is sufficiently consistent and strong to cate-
gorize various environmental exposures as linked to different types of
cancer, though the specific carcinogens and the mechanisms of cancer
induction have not always been definitely determined (see chart). The
chemical carcinogens—for example, ovarian hormones, testosterone,

MAJOR CAUSES OF CANCER

Known or Probable Causes	Possible Causes	Cancer
Tobacco		Lung, bladder, pancreas, kidney, stomach
Tobacco and alcohol		Oral cavity, esophagus, larynx, pharynx
Hepatitis viruses, alcohol	Tobacco	Liver
Animal fat and low fiber		Colon or rectum
Ovarian hormones		Breast
Testosterone		Prostate
Estrogen		Uterus
	Papilloma viruses	Cervix
Ovulation		Ovary
X rays		Leukemia, brain tumors
Ultraviolet		Skin cancer, melanoma
HTLV-I		Non-Hodgkin's lymphoma, adult T-cell lymphoma

SOURCE: Adapted from table in B. E. Henderson, R. K. Ross, and M. C. Pike, "Toward the Primary Prevention of Cancer," *Science* 254 (1991).

estrogens—may cause cancer by increasing the rate of cell proliferation. The physical carcinogens—for example, X rays, ultraviolet radiation—may cause cancer by direct damage to the DNA itself. The chemicals from tobacco and their metabolic products may combine both effects.

The acceleration of cell division appears to be the more important of the two mechanisms; it results in increased rates of mutation of the protooncogenes and tumor-suppressor genes. It is believed that removal of the carcinogen at almost any stage of the multistep process of carcinogenesis can interfere with or deter the development of the disease.

TOBACCO

Smoking is one factor that has definitely been correlated with increased cancer risk. Tobacco alone, or in combination with alcohol, is now the most important cause of cancer, the culprit behind approximately one of every three cancer cases in the United States. These include cancers of the lung, oral cavity, esophagus, pharynx, larynx, pancreas, and bladder. Smokeless tobacco—chewing tobacco and snuff—is a well-established cause of cancers of the oral cavity. As recently as 1985, approximately twelve million individuals, many of them adolescents, were estimated to be using smokeless tobacco (Henderson 1991). Fortunately, preventive strategies are apparently succeeding in reducing the popularity of tobacco.

DIET

Dietary factors have been evaluated as a possible cause of cancer and as a way of preventing cancer. We know this mainly from epidemiological studies (analyses of patterns in different populations), but the underlying mechanisms for these effects have not yet been elucidated. In 1977, E. L. Wynder and G. B. Gori analyzed differences between cancer mortality rates in the United States and in those countries with the lowest rates and concluded that 40 percent of cancers in men and up to 60 percent in women could be accounted for by dietary factors. Similar analyses by R. Doll and R. Peto in 1981 estimated that a 35 percent reduction in cancer deaths might be achieved if diets were properly modified, although they cautioned that such estimates are speculative (in Heber 1984). The specific sites of cancer most likely to be affected are the stomach, large intestine, uterus, and breast.

Cancers of the stomach, colon, and rectum accounted for 17 percent of all new cancers in the United States in 1990. While stomach cancer is known to be caused by tobacco, salt and food preservatives are also key factors. The decline in the incidence of stomach cancer throughout the world in recent years has been associated with a decline in the salting and pickling of food and the simultaneous increase in the consumption of fresh fruits and vegetables. A strong correlation between stomach cancer and the consumption of preserved and highly salty food has been observed in many populations throughout the world. The corrosive effects of large amounts of salt and pickling compounds upon the stomach lining lead to cell injury and death, followed by regeneration of the mucosal cells, accompanied by an increase in genetic alterations.

With colon and rectal cancers, the important factors are dietary fat and fiber. Epidemiological studies indicate a relationship between animal fat in red meats and colon and rectal cancer. Since an individual's total fat consumption is correlated with the consumption of animal fat, it has been difficult to sort out precisely the kind of fat (total fat, saturated fat, vegetable fat) that is most closely linked to cancer. The most recent studies indicate that the consumption of animal fat in red meats (beef, lamb, and pork) is more closely correlated with colon cancer than the consumption of dairy products with their fat content. These studies also suggest that a 50 percent decrease in the consumption of animal fat would result in approximately the same reduction in colon cancer risk (Henderson 1991).

The mechanisms by which fat causes colon and rectal cancer is unknown, but we do know that when rodents are fed diets high in saturated fat, the lining of the colon becomes inflamed and cells are killed and lost, leading to a compensatory regeneration of the injured cells. An increase in cell proliferation sets the stage for alterations in protooncogenes and tumor-suppressor genes.

Although some investigators have revealed associations between fat consumption and the incidence of cancer of the breast, prostate, ovaries, and uterus, these correlations are not as consistent as those for colon and rectal cancer. In some population studies that compared survival rates of breast cancer patients in the United States— where fat consumption is about 37 percent of total calories—with those in Japan—where fat consumption is only 11 percent of total calories—the survival rates in Japan were significantly and consistently greater (Morrison et al. 1976; Makita et al. 1990; Chlebowski et al. 1991).

Excess caloric intake leading to obesity, rather than the composition of the diet, seems to be important in hormone-related cancers. Obesity is a known risk factor in uterine cancer, and obesity in childhood may lead to early puberty, an important risk factor in breast cancer.

In addition to a diet high in fat, a diet low in fiber is also associated in some studies with an increased risk of colon cancer (Henderson 1991). This association is not as well established as that between fat and colon cancer (for instance, it has been reported that women with the highest consumption of animal fat and the lowest consumption of crude fiber had the highest risk of colon cancer). While most of the evidence suggests the protective effect of fiber, the specific source of this effect (cereals, vegetables, fruits) has not been delineated.

It has been proposed that dietary fiber reduces cancer by increasing the proportion of water in the intestinal contents and decreasing transit time through the colon, thus diluting the effect of carcinogens (such as the metabolic products of fats and bile acids) and reducing the length of time they are in contact with the cells lining the colon. Dietary fiber has been found to reduce the level of circulating estrogens as well.

Alcohol, alone and together with tobacco, increases the risk of cancers of the mouth, pharynx, larynx, esophagus, and liver. All types of alcoholic beverages—beer, wine, and various distilled whiskeys—are equally likely to increase the risks of these cancers. Alcohol intake has also been linked to cancers of the colon, rectum, and breast, but here the causal relationship is less significant.

Many natural mutagens and carcinogens have been found in a variety of foods in the diet, ranging from urethanes in mustard to a fermentation product in beer, yogurt, bread, and other foods. Bruce N. Ames of the University of California, Berkeley, who developed a widely used test for the detection of mutagens, has written extensively about dietary carcinogens and concludes that "nature is not benign." In fact, these carcinogens are more abundant, more potent, and more likely to cause cancer than are pesticides or food additives. On a more positive note, many foods do contain anticarcinogens that act as protective factors against other natural and environmental risk factors.

Other examples of carcinogens in food are toxins produced by molds, such as aflatoxin, which contaminates corn, soybeans, peanuts, and rice. A potent carcinogen, aflatoxin has been shown to cause liver cancer as a result of a specific mutation of the p53 tumor-suppressor gene. Nitropyrenes in charred meat and fish may also cause alteration in genes associated with carcinogenesis. Suggested modifications of the diet that may lower the risk of cancer will be discussed later in the chapter.

HORMONES

Hormones are also associated with certain cancers. They appeared to play a role in approximately one-third of all new cancer cases in 1990 (Henderson 1991). For example, the long-term cumulative effects of estrogen and progesterone in women who have early onset of menstrual periods and late menopause are important risk factors for breast cancer. The risk is reduced 10 to 20 percent for each year regular menstrual cycles are delayed. Women who stop menstruating before the age of forty-five, either naturally or surgically, face half the risk of breast cancer of women who continue to menstruate to age fifty-five.

Women with breast cancer have higher estrogen levels than healthy women, and estrogen levels are higher in populations of women who have higher rates of breast cancer. American women develop breast cancer four to six times as often as Japanese women; this can be explained, in part, by the higher estrogen levels and earlier age of menstruation of the Americans.

The use of estrogen replacement in postmenopausal women results in approximately a 10 percent increase in the risk of breast cancer for each year of such therapy. When both estrogen and progesterone are used by postmenopausal women, the risk is even larger, though this combined supplement lowers the risk of uterine cancer. This statistic can be explained by the increase in breast cell proliferation when progesterone levels are high.

In view of these findings, it might be asked whether pregnancy increases the risk of breast cancer, because both estrogen and progesterone levels are elevated during pregnancy. The association is a complex one. The high hormone levels during pregnancy cause not only breast cell proliferation but also cell differentiation, thereby reducing the progression to unregulated cancer cells. Further, breast-feeding with the stimulation of lactation appears to have a protective effect, possibly because of the cessation of ovulation and the resulting progesterone deficiency.

Uterine cancer is caused by the cumulative effects of estrogens in the absence of progesterone. Estrogen causes endometrial (uterine) cells to divide, but the simultaneous presence of progesterone can suppress such mitotic activity. Estrogen stimulation "unopposed" by progesterone increases the risk of uterine cancer. Postmenopausal women in the 1970s who took large doses of estrogen alone experienced three times as much uterine cancer for each five years of treatment as untreated women (Henderson 1991). Reducing the dose of estrogen and adding progesterone reversed this trend.

These observations support the concept that estrogen-induced proliferation of endometrial cells increases the risk of this cancer. Additional evidence comes from the use of combination-type oral contraceptive pills that contain estrogen and progesterone, which reduce uterine cancer risk. The pills are taken for twenty-one days, followed by seven days of no treatment. Thus the endometrial cells are exposed to estrogen unopposed by progesterone for only seven days, and the blood estrogen is low during this time. Young women who have taken the pill for five years have an incidence of endometrial cancer about 55 percent less than nonusers (Henderson 1991). Finally, obesity in postmenopausal women increases the risk of uterine cancer because fat tissues produce some estrogens, and postmenopausal women are no longer producing progesterone to counteract them.

Prostate cancer is most likely also related to the long-term cumulative exposure to hormones, in this case testosterone and possibly estrogen. In the body, testosterone, after enzymatic conversion to dihydrotestosterone, enhances mitotic activity in the prostate. Black males have the highest incidence of prostate cancer in the world. Blood testosterone and estrogen levels in young black men are higher than in young white men and are thought to account for the twofold greater incidence of prostate cancer later in life. Additionally, black women have markedly higher blood levels of testosterone and estrogen during early pregnancy than do white women, and it has been suggested that these high levels may contribute to the high incidence of prostate cancer in black male offspring. The reason for these high levels of testosterone and estrogen in black populations is unknown. In contrast to black men, Japanese men have the lowest rates of prostate cancer in the world. This may be due to differences in testosterone metabolism in Japanese men, but little data are available to support this possibility.

OTHER CAUSES

A number of other factors, including drugs, medical and dental X rays, ultraviolet light, and chronic irritation or trauma, are associated with cancer. It is estimated that these extraneous factors cause about 20 percent of all cancers (Henderson 1991). Medical interventions by various drugs, diagnostic or therapeutic X rays, and other agents (see appendix, table 8) represent a small contribution to the total number of cancers, which are potentially preventable. For example, the initial type of estrogen replacement therapy without progesterone increased the risk of both uterine and breast cancer. *In utero* exposure to the synthetic estrogen diethylstilbestrol was associated with adenocarcinomas of the vagina in adolescent and young adult women. Other drugs, including phenacetin, and diuretics, appear to be carcinogenic for the lower urinary tract and kidney, respectively. Regrettably, some chemotherapeutic drugs used to treat childhood cancer, such as cyclophosphamide, may cause second cancers in long-term survivors.

Individuals exposed to high radiation doses, such as atomic bomb survivors or those receiving radiation therapy for specific health problems, are at risk of leukemia and many solid tumors. The relationship between low-dose diagnostic radiation and various cancers is controversial, but it is estimated that 16 percent of all leukemias in the United States have been caused by diagnostic radiation (Henderson 1991).

Physical irritation or trauma has also been associated with specific cancers. For instance, 80 percent of patients with gallbladder cancer have gallstones. Head trauma may lead to brain tumors and asbestos to lung cancers, especially mesotheliomas. In these examples it is proposed that the irritation of the gallstones, trauma, or asbestos fibers leads to cell injury followed by cell proliferation during the repair of damaged tissue. It is during the active cell division that alterations of the crucial protooncogenes and tumor-suppressor genes may take place.

Occupational cancers—those caused by exposure to carcinogenic agents in the workplace—are estimated to account for less than 4 percent of cancers in the United States (see appendix, table 7). Lung cancers caused by the major offender, asbestos, seem to have peaked in the mid-1980s. The saga of cancers induced by asbestos is like that of the cancers that appeared in atomic bomb survivors many years after 1945. In the case of asbestos, World War II shipyard workers were heavily exposed to this agent and developed lung mesotheliomas many years later.

The role of viruses in human cancer is also important (see chapter 1 and appendix, table 4). The strongest cause-and-effect relationship is between the hepatitis B virus and hepatocellular carcinoma, a cancer that is extremely common in parts of Asia and Africa but rare in the United States. Strong evidence also links certain human papillomaviruses with cervical cancer, and the human T-cell lymphotropic virus type I to adult T-cell lymphomas. The Epstein-Barr virus plays an important role, along with immunological defects, in Burkitt's and other highly malignant lymphomas.

Besides viruses, the first bacterium discovered to play a role in human cancer is the *Helicobacter pylori*. This microorganism is a major cause of gastritis in some parts of the world and has been associated with stomach cancer, possibly through the same mechanism described previously for salt, namely, injury to the cells lining the stomach followed by cell proliferation during the regeneration process.

The major causes of cancer, such as tobacco, fat, alcohol, obesity, and ultraviolet light, are clearly associated with lifestyle and not with the environment in general. Unfortunately, there is a widespread misperception that environmental pollution is the major cause of cancer. Fortunately, individual practices that are its major causes can be amended.

Lifestyle Changes to Prevent Cancer

We are now armed with sufficient information to aid in the prevention of a majority of the most common human cancers—those associated with personal choices of lifestyle (see chart).

Strenuous efforts to reduce *cigarette smoking* have been undertaken, and some headway has been made. More efforts must be aimed at adolescents, especially girls, and the entire Third World. Also targeted for behavioral modification must be the use of *smokeless tobacco* (chewing tobacco and snuff), again, especially in adolescents. The general public is now incensed about passive smoking, and tighter restrictions on smoking on airplanes and indeed in all public places are being sought.

CAUSES OF CANCER	PREVENTIVE MEASURES
TOBACCO	Stop smoking cigarettes, cigars, and pipes. Stop use of smokeless tobacco. Take action to avoid and curtail passive smoking.
DIETARY FACTORS TOTAL FAT	Replace high-fat red meats in diet with low-fat dairy products, lean meat, poultry, fish, and beans.
HIGHLY SALTED AND PRESERVED FOODS	Reduce intake of salt-cured, smoked, and nitrate-cured foods, such as hot dogs, ham, bacon, fish, and charred foods.
LOW INTAKE OF FIBER	Increase fiber intake to 20–30 grams per day, eat more varied grains, fruits, vegetables.

	Increase consumption of fresh fruits and vegetables that are rich in beta-carotene and vitamins A, C, and E. Increase consumption of cereals and whole grains, legumes.
ALCOHOL	Reduce consumption of alcohol. Substitute nonalcoholic forms of such beverages as beer.
OBESITY	Reduce consumption of high-calorie food and make efforts to control weight.
SEDENTARY LIFE	Exercise regularly, at least 3 times a week for 30 minutes.
SUNLIGHT	Avoid sun, especially during midday hours; use sunscreen and wear protective clothing.
OCCUPATIONAL EXPOSURE	Avoid exposure to cancer-causing agents: asbestos, benzene, carbon tetrachloride, soots, tars, chromium, nickel and cadmium compounds, vinyl chloride. See appendix, tables 6 and 7.
MEDICAL PROCEDURES OR PRESCRIBED DRUGS	When possible, avoid or reduce exposure to diagnostic or therapeutic X rays and to various drugs such as estrogens and phenacetin.
GENETIC BACKGROUND	Members of families with strong history of cancer, such as those with Li-Fraumeni syndrome, should seek expert medical consultation on appropriate measures (mammography, physical examinations, eye examinations) to detect cancer in early stage.
VIRUSES	Hepatitis B. Vaccine to control liver cancer in high-risk areas of Asia and Africa. Effective vaccines against papillomaviruses, HTLV-I, and HIV can theoretically be produced.

Excessive alcohol consumption is yet another cause of cancer, especially when combined with tobacco. Fortunately, alcohol consumption has decreased in the United States in response to heightened public awareness of the dangers of drunk driving and alcoholism and all substance abuse. The availability of nonalcoholic beers may also reduce alcohol consumption. These hopeful developments, if continued, will reduce not only alcoholism but also the alcohol-induced cancers, notably those of the colon and other segments of the gastrointestinal tract.

Increasing *physical activity* promotes bowel contraction, which speeds the fecal stream and reduces the time colonic cells are exposed to any carcinogens in waste, thereby reducing the risk of colon cancer—one of the many reasons for advocating a program of physical exercise.

Excessive *exposure to sunlight* has made Australia the country with the highest incidence of melanoma, but it has increased in both incidence and mortality in the United States as well. Other, less dangerous skin cancers, such as basal-cell and squamous-cell, account for about 600,000 new cancer cases per year in the United States. The public has become increasingly aware that the pleasant experience of sunbathing can be a direct cause of skin cancer, as well as premature aging of the skin. Besides being a recreational hazard, sunlight is also an occupational hazard, especially for farmers and sailors. The use of protective sunscreens and protective clothing must be strongly encouraged.

Medical procedures and prescribed drugs that result in disorders or disease are termed *iatrogenic*. Only a few cancers are now caused by such agents, and they are mostly preventable. The radiation exposure from modern X-ray equipment is much lower than it used to be. The addition of progesterone to estrogen replacement therapy for postmenopausal women has reduced the incidence of uterine cancer. Unfortunately, some chemotherapeutic drugs, such as cyclophosphamide, used to treat and often cure childhood cancers are now known to cause second cancers years later.

In recent years, more attention has been (and should continue to be) focused on *occupational exposure* to carcinogens, alerting workers to the hazards and advocating the use of masks and other protective devices.

The effect of *diet modification* to reduce cancer risk is an area of active investigation and increasing importance, amenable to individual control. The most prudent course is to eat a balanced diet with an increased intake of yellow fruits, dark green vegetables, and high-fiber whole grains and breads and cereals, and to decrease consumption of fat, particularly animal fat. Although investigations on diet and cancer are still in the preliminary stages, researchers in this field are changing their own diets in the modest ways recommended. The results have been encouraging enough to warrant their compliance.

Recent studies suggest that a 50 percent reduction in the level of dietary animal fat alone could cut in half the incidence of the second most common cancer in the United States, colon and rectal. A balanced diet in which fat is restricted to 20 percent of total calories is proposed in a planned clinical study that should further delineate the role of fat in cancer. Similar studies in women with breast cancer or at high risk for developing it are also projected. The correlation of reduced fat intake with reduced incidence of hormone-related cancers—breast, prostate, uterine, ovarian—has not been consistent.

Avoiding *obesity* by engaging in a moderate exercise program and limiting caloric intake has been suggested as more important in lowering the risk of hormone-related cancers than reduced fat intake, though the two factors may be related.

Although it has been suggested that Americans double their intake of *fiber*, to 20 to 30 grams daily, there is as yet no conclusive evidence that lack of fiber plays a significant part in carcinogenesis. Fiber represents a heterogeneous group of plant substances that are resistant to digestion, thereby decreasing the transit time of body waste, including many carcinogens, through the colon. Because there are many different types of fiber, it is prudent to consume a variety of high-fiber foods: whole-grain breads and cereals, fruits, legumes, nuts, and vegetables such as broccoli, cauliflower, brussels sprouts, and cabbage. A large-scale clinical study designed to evaluate the effectiveness of such a diet in lowering the incidence of adenomatous polyps, a condition that can lead to colon cancer, is under way at the National Cancer Institute.

Food is also a source of anticarcinogens, which act by hindering the formation of carcinogens in the body or by counteracting the effects of the carcinogens themselves. Among these *micronutrients* (so called because they are believed to be required in much smaller amounts than carbohydrates, proteins, and fats) are a group called retinoids— beta-carotene and Vitamin A—found in yellow vegetables and fruit; Vitamin C, found in broccoli, citrus fruits, tomatoes, and strawberries; and Vitamin E, in whole grains, vegetable oils, and vegetables. See the section on chemoprevention for a discussion of the clinical trials that are under way to determine the effect of these micronutrients on cancer incidence.

The talents and resources expended by the medical profession have often been directed at medical treatment rather than prevention of disease. Cancer is an outstanding example of this tendency. Neither early diagnosis nor improved therapy is likely to reduce the incidence of cancer. These measures can, of course, reduce mortality rates in patients with cancer, but they have no effect on the numbers of new cases that are diagnosed annually.

According to Denis Burkitt, the English physician who identified Burkitt's lymphoma, a whole spectrum of diseases rampant in modern Western society is caused by the new environment into which we have plunged and for which we are not genetically adapted (Burkitt 1991). Many of the major diseases in the modern West, among both blacks and whites, are rare in all Third World countries and were uncommon even in the United States until after World War I. These findings imply that such diseases must be due not to our genetic background but to our modern lifestyle, to environmental or behavioral change. This conclusion in turn suggests that they must be potentially preventable.

People in Western society have made more changes in lifestyle and eating habits in the last 200 to 300 years than in the previous 20,000 years. Our ancestors were hunter-gatherers for many thousands of years. They ate mainly foods that contained starch and fiber, but little animal fat. It is to that type of culture to which we are genetically coded, and our genes have scarcely altered since those prehistoric days. The first major change in lifestyle occurred during the Agricultural Revolution about 10,000 years ago, but this change was minor compared to the enormous changes associated with the Industrial Revolution about 200 years ago. The major dietary changes that followed the Industrial Revolution included a reduction in starch foods and fiber and a great increase in animal fats, salt, and sugar. The contrasts between ancient and Third World peasant diets are small compared with the contrasts between these and modern foods (see chart).

Burkitt contends that we are putting modern fast foods into Stone Age bodies. And, in fact, our modern lifestyle is associated with a shocking list of diseases: coronary heart disease, the most common cause of death; diabetes, the most common endocrine disease; appendicitis, the most common abdominal emergency; colon and rectal cancers, the second most common cause of cancer death (after lung

Estimated Components of Ancient, Third World, and Modern Western Diets

Component	Ancient	Third World	Modern Western
Starch	60%	60%	20%
Sugar	Minimal	Minimal	20%
Protein	20%	15%	15%
Fat	20%	15%	45%
Fiber	50–100 grams/day	50–100 grams/day	Less than 20 grams/day

Source: Adapted from table in D. Burkitt, "Are Our Commonest Diseases Preventable?" *The Pharos* 54 (1991): 19–21.

cancer); breast cancer, the most common cancer in women; and prostate cancer, the third most common cause of death in men.

The wide acceptance of this concept has led specialists in different branches of medicine to recommend similar dietary regimes for the prevention of diseases within their specialties. The cardiologist, the diabetologist, and the gastroenterologist all recommend an increased consumption of fiber and a reduced intake of fat. Oncologists stress the causative role of fat and the protective role of dietary fiber in cancer of the colon and the rectum and possibly the breast. The type of diet that is least likely to cause all of these diseases—cancer, heart disease, and diabetes—is one that provides a high proportion of whole-grain cereals, vegetables, and fruits. This diet would also provide most of its animal protein in poultry and fish (but not smoked or grilled) and would include very few eggs or dairy products and little sugar. Finally, the diet should be sufficiently restricted to avoid obesity.

People who are aware that this type of diet might simultaneously protect against a number of major diseases should be more eager to comply with it. Physicians and other professionals should explain to patients that our genetic constitution is tailor-made for an environment of many thousand years ago. While our genes have not changed much, the environment, especially our diet, has changed drastically. The only way to regain concordance between our genes and our lifestyle is to alter the latter toward one for which we are genetically endowed.

New Preventive Measures

SCREENING FOR GENES

Classical epidemiology has been used in the past to identify groups of people at high risk for developing cancer. Newer methods focusing on the genes involved in carcinogenesis have made possible a different approach, one that attempts to identify individual cancer risk and answer the question, What is *my* risk of getting cancer?

One set of such predictions comes from screening individuals for one of a few defective genes—Rb, p53, or FAP (found in *f*amilial *a*denomatous *p*olyposis)—and determining individual cancer susceptibility. Even if such a defective gene is detected, the road to take is far from clear. As we have pointed out, cancer is a multistep process involving the alteration of several genes, and the presence of one defective gene does not invariably lead to cancer. When the gene detected is an Rb gene, the course seems clearer because about 95 percent of those carrying the defective gene develop retinoblastoma by the age of five. Regular eye examinations to detect signs of cancer, followed by noninvasive treatment, result in almost 100 percent survival, without the loss of the eye.

But other genes, like the mutation in the p53 gene in Li-Fraumeni patients—a group highly susceptible to at least six types of cancer, which they develop as children or young adults—present a much more complicated picture both medically and ethically.

A screening test for colon and rectal cancer was recently described based on the detection of a mutated *ras* oncogene in tumor cells shed in the patient's stool. Such a noninvasive technique could be used to screen asymptomatic individuals who are at high risk for this common form of cancer. In fact, it was recently suggested that such techniques could be applied to screening for a tumor-suppressor gene found in the FAP gene at an early stage on the road to colon cancer.

MOLECULAR EPIDEMIOLOGY

Inherited genetic defects represent only a small part of the problem. Most cancers are believed to be caused by exposure to environmental carcinogens. The new field of molecular epidemiology attempts to find people who are at high risk because of their exposure to such carcinogens and to determine exactly what the biochemical effects of these carcinogens are. Individuals vary considerably in their response to carcinogens. For example, only one in ten smokers develops lung cancer. Instead of screening for mutated genes in inaccessible tissues like liver and lung, investigators are seeking biochemical "surrogates," substances formed as the result of an individual's exposure to the carcinogen that can be easily assayed in the urine or blood.

One such surrogate is an adduct formed between the DNA and the carcinogen, which may result in mutations that give rise to cancer. People in China and West Africa, where exposure to the carcinogen aflatoxin is high, show elevated concentrations of the aflatoxin adduct. Another study shows that exposure to polycyclic aromatic hydrocarbons (PAHs), potent carcinogens, by iron foundry workers in Finland and coke-oven workers in Poland, can be correlated with adduct formation.

Interestingly, increases in this adduct have also been found in people living in highly polluted areas of Poland, creating a suggestive link between environmental pollution and cancer. There is cautious optimism that these biochemical markers can be correlated with individual cancer risk and used to alert people who are at high risk.

CHEMOPREVENTION

Identifying individuals at high risk raises the question of what kinds of preventive measures are available, aside from being watched closely by their physicians. A strategy called *chemoprevention* is designed to fill this role by using drugs or dietary changes to ward off cancer development.

The National Cancer Institute is currently sponsoring some forty trials involving 77,000 people to study the most common cancers—lung, colon/rectal, and breast. These individuals are not cancer patients but healthy people who are at high risk for cancer, some with precancerous conditions and some who have had cancer but are now disease-free. The agents being tested must be free of toxic side effects because these healthy people may use them for many years. The substances used are vitamins (such as A, C, or E), high-fiber foods, or drugs that have been widely used for years, such as aspirin, ibuprofen, or calcium carbonate. One trial will include 17,000 men at high risk for developing lung cancer from smoking or asbestos exposure, who will be treated with daily doses of beta-carotene and Vitamin A.

There have been preliminary studies in the United States and Europe indicating that beta-carotene, a precursor of Vitamin A, results in a consistent, moderate decrease in the incidence of lung cancer. A large study of 19,000 women who smoke will be given Vitamin E along with beta-carotene, to determine the effect on lung cancer risk. A summary of some of these trials appears in the accompanying chart.

Selected Agents in Chemoprevention Trials

Drug	Cancer	Mechanism of Action
Retinoids (Vitamin A)	Skin, lung, breast, cervix	Induces cell maturation and inhibits proliferation
Beta-carotene	Lung, cervix, skin	Similar to retinoids
Calcium carbonate/calcium lactate	Colon	Binds bile acids; decreases their proliferative effects
DFMO (difluoromethyl-ornithine)	Colon	Antiproliferative; blocks polyamine synthesis
Ibuprofen	Colon	Anti-inflammatory
α-Tocopherol (Vitamin E)	Colon	Antioxidant
Tamoxifen	Breast	Anti-inflammatory, antiestrogen

SOURCE: From table in J. Marx, "Zeroing In on Individual Cancer Risk," *Science* 253 (1991): 253. Copyright © by the American Association for the Advancement of Science.

Such a strategy has long been championed by Linus Pauling, who has argued that Vitamin C can prevent not only the common cold but also cancer. There is some inconclusive evidence that Vitamin C has a protective effect against several epithelial cancers, such as those of the oral cavity, pharynx, and larynx. Several clinical trials are under way to determine whether beta-carotene and vitamins C and E, which trap reactive oxygen compounds in the cell, may help patients at elevated risk of cancer of the lung, esophagus, colon, and skin. The data, although inconclusive, also suggest a protective effect. The element selenium, found in foods, has also been touted as having a preventive effect against cancer. Unpublished data from studies in China suggest that this is not the case, however.

A breast cancer prevention trial using tamoxifen is being carried out on 16,000 women at high risk for developing that cancer. This antiestrogenic drug has been used in breast cancer patients after surgery in an effort to block growth of any remaining cancer cells. Tamoxifen acts by blocking estrogen, the hormone that stimulates the growth of breast cells. Currently several families of drugs are also being developed that block testosterone activity. These agents might one day be used to prevent prostate cancer.

The large number of chemoprevention trials under way or projected attests to the enthusiasm and excitement generated by this new emphasis on the prevention of cancer.

In this book, we have distilled vast quantities of information and disconnected facts to help explain the mystery of cancer. It is of interest to note that in 1802, a group of leading English physicians asked thirteen questions about cancer. In the appendix we have listed the questions and attempted to answer them. Although much work still needs to be done, it is abundantly clear that some simple concepts are emerging from the previous chaos. One of the most encouraging of these is that the preponderance of cancer is caused by environmental factors over which we have some measure of control and about which we are learning to make more judicious choices. We have entered a new era, when scientists can study ways to prevent cancer as well as develop more effective weapons to treat it. Progression along these lines holds the promise of controlling this frightening scourge of mankind.

APPENDIX

Cancer Centers in the United States

COMPREHENSIVE CENTERS

These are the major components of the National Cancer Institute's network of cancer resource facilities. They must meet specific criteria to be designated as regional and national hubs for cancer research, training, and treatment.

1. University of Alabama, Birmingham, Alabama.
2. University of Arizona, Tucson, Arizona.
3. University of Southern California (USC), Los Angeles.
4. University of California, Jonsson Comprehensive Cancer Center (UCLA), Los Angeles.
5. Yale School of Medicine, New Haven, Connecticut.
6. Sylvester Comprehensive Cancer Center, University of Miami Medical School, Miami, Florida.
7. Johns Hopkins Oncology Center, Baltimore, Maryland.
8. Dana-Farber Cancer Institute, Boston, Massachusetts.
9. Comprehensive Cancer Center of Metropolitan Detroit, Wayne State University, Detroit, Michigan.
10. Mayo Comprehensive Cancer Center, Mayo Clinic, Rochester, Minnesota.
11. Norris Cotton Cancer Center, Dartmouth-Hitchcock Medical Center, Hanover, New Hampshire.
12. Memorial Sloan-Kettering Cancer Center, New York, New York.
13. Roswell Park Memorial Institute, Buffalo, New York.
14. Columbia University Cancer Center, College of Physicians and Surgeons, New York, New York.
15. Duke University, Durham, North Carolina.
16. Lineberger Comprehensive Cancer Center, University of North Carolina School of Medicine, Chapel Hill.
17. Wake Forest University, Bowman Gray School of Medicine, Winston-Salem, North Carolina.
18. Arthur G. James Cancer Hospital, Ohio State University, Columbus.

19. Fox Chase Cancer Center, Philadelphia, Pennsylvania.
20. University of Pennsylvania, Philadelphia.
21. University of Pittsburgh, Pittsburgh, Pennsylvania.
22. M. D. Anderson Cancer Center, University of Texas, Houston.
23. Fred Hutchinson Cancer Research Center, Seattle, Washington.
24. University of Wisconsin, Madison.

CLINICAL CENTERS

These facilities conduct research and treat patients.

1. University of California, San Diego.
2. City of Hope National Medical Center, Beckman Research Institute, Duarte, California.
3. University of Colorado Health Sciences Center, Denver.
4. Lombardi Cancer Research Center, Georgetown University Medical Center, Washington, D.C.
5. University of Chicago Cancer Research Center, Chicago, Illinois.
6. University of Michigan Cancer Center, Ann Arbor.
7. Albert Einstein College of Medicine, Bronx, New York.
8. New York University Medical Center, New York, New York.
9. University of Rochester Cancer Center, Rochester, New York.
10. Case Western Reserve University, Ireland Cancer Center, Cleveland, Ohio.
11. Brown University, Roger Williams Medical Center, Providence, Rhode Island.
12. St. Jude Children's Research Hospital, Memphis, Tennessee.
13. Institute for Cancer Research and Care, San Antonio, Texas.
14. Utah Regional Cancer Center, University of Utah Medical Center, Salt Lake City.
15. Vermont Regional Cancer Center, University of Vermont, Burlington.
16. Massey Cancer Center, Medical College of Virginia, Virginia Commonwealth University, Richmond.

BASIC CENTERS

These centers primarily conduct laboratory research. They rarely treat patients.

1. La Jolla Cancer Research Foundation, La Jolla, California.
2. Armand Hammer Center for Cancer Biology, Salk Institute, San Diego, California.
3. California Institute of Technology, Biology Division, Pasadena, California.
4. Purdue University, West Lafayette, Indiana.
5. Jackson Laboratory, Bar Harbor, Maine.
6. Worcester Foundation for Experimental Biology, Shrewsbury, Massachusetts.
7. Center for Cancer Research, Massachusetts Institute of Technology, Cambridge.
8. Eppley Institute, University of Nebraska, Omaha.
9. Cold Spring Harbor Laboratory, Cold Spring Harbor, New York.
10. New York University Medical Center, New York, New York.
11. American Health Foundation, New York, New York.
12. Wistar Institute Cancer Center, Philadelphia, Pennsylvania.
13. Fels Research Institute, Temple University School of Medicine, Philadelphia, Pennsylvania.
14. University of Virginia Medical Center, Charlottesville.
15. McArdle Laboratory for Cancer Research, University of Wisconsin, Madison.

CONSORTIUM CENTERS

Made up of two or more institutions, these centers operate cancer control and research programs.

1. Illinois Cancer Council, Chicago.
2. Drew-Meharry-Morehouse Consortium Cancer Center, Nashville, Tennessee.

Current Answers to Some Old Questions
About Cancer

Two hundred years ago, a group of leading English physicians formed the Institution for Investigating the Nature and Cure of Cancer. In 1802, they proposed thirteen questions about the disease. It is of interest to pose these questions again and attempt to answer them.

1. *What are the diagnostic signs of cancer?*
    Signs of cancer, such as masses or ulcers detected on physical examination, have been recognized and described since ancient Egyptian times. Chapters 9–18 describe the signs of the ten most common cancers in the United States.

2. *Does any alteration take place in the structure of a part, preceding that more obvious change which is called cancer? If there does, what is the nature of that alteration?*
    Many types of structural alterations in the form of benign lesions precede and develop into cancer. Polyps and adenomas (tumors of the glands) of the colon progress into cancer after a series of molecular alterations in oncogenes and tumor-suppressor genes, as discussed in chapter 5.

3. *Is cancer always an original and primary disease, or may other diseases degenerate into cancer?*
    Although cancer is usually a primary disease, certain other diseases, such as Xeroderma pigmentosa of the skin and cervical warts, regularly degenerate into cancer.

4. *Are there any proofs of cancer being a hereditary disease?*
    Yes. The role of heredity in certain cancers, such as breast cancer and retinoblastoma, is described in this book.

5. *Are there any proofs of cancer being a contagious disease?*
    For years, cancer was not considered to be "catching" among humans. The discovery of HTLV-I in 1980, however, indicated that it could spread from one individual to another and cause adult T-cell leukemia. Further, the hepatitis B virus, Epstein-Barr virus, and papillomaviruses are infectious agents that are co-factors in certain cancers.

6. *Is there any well-marked relation between cancer and other diseases? If there be, what are those diseases to which it bears the nearest resemblance in its origin, progress, and termination?*

   Yes. Patients with diseases of the immune system regularly develop lymphoma. Also, patients with organ transplants who receive immunosuppressive drugs and patients with AIDS sometimes develop B-cell lymphomas. Other examples are known.

7. *May cancer be regarded at any period, or under any circumstances, merely as a local disease? Or does the existence of cancer in one part afford a presumption that there is a tendency to a similar morbid alteration in other parts of the animal system?*

   Most cancers can be considered potentially capable of metastatic spread, although some, such as basal-cell cancer of the skin, often remain localized.

8. *Has climate, or local situation, any influence in rendering the human constitution more or less liable to cancer under any form or in any part?*

   Yes. Excessive exposure to the sun in temperate zones leads to melanomas. Malaria in equatorial Africa apparently renders African children at risk for Burkitt's lymphoma. A liver cancer, hepatocellular carcinoma, is extremely common in parts of China and Africa, where chronic infection with hepatitis B virus is prevalent and aflatoxin contaminates food.

9. *Is there a particular temperament of body more liable to be affected with cancer than others? And, if there be, what is the temperament?*

   Some behavioral scientists believe that psychological stresses render some individuals more susceptible than others to cancer.

10. *Are brute creatures subject to any disease resembling cancer in the human subject?*

    Yes. Many types of cancer have been detected, especially in older animals, in every species of animal that has been carefully studied.

11. *Is there any period of life absolutely exempt from the attack of this disease?*
No. Cancer has even been known to develop in fetuses before birth. Although it can develop in individuals at any age, it is much more common in older people.

12. *Are the lymphatic glands ever affected primarily in cancer?*
Yes. Lymphomas can develop in the lymph nodes.

13. *Is cancer under any circumstances susceptible of a natural cure?*
Yes. Certain cancers, such as neuroblastomas (tumors of primitive nerve cells in children), can on rare occasion regress spontaneously. Of a recent report of 112 cancers that regressed spontaneously, 25 were neuroblastomas, 14 were choriocarcinomas (tumors of fetal cells), 11 were kidney carcinomas, 10 were melanomas, and 9 were sarcomas (Elverson 1964).

TABLE 1 *History of Chemical Carcinogenesis*

Year	Chemical Carcinogen	Investigator
1775	*Chimney soot* associated with scrotal cancer in chimney sweeps.	Sir P. Pott
1895	*Aniline dye, 2-naphthylamine,* associated with bladder cancer in factory workers.	L. Rehn
1915	*Coal tar* application produces skin carcinomas in rabbits.	K. Yamagawa
1938	*Creosote oil* enhances the induction by benzopyrene of skin tumors in the mouse.	M. Shear
1941	Co-carcinogenesis: initiation by *coal tar* and promotion by *croton oil.*	I. Berenblum
1950	Causal relationship shown between *tobacco smoking* and lung cancer.	E. Wynder E. Graham M. Levin
1950/1964	Health hazards of *cigarette smoking.*	Sir R. Doll Sir A. B. Hill
1961	*Aflatoxin,* a toxin of a fungus that contaminates some foods (such as peanuts and grains) shown to cause liver cancer in Asia and Africa.	M. C. Lancaster
1976	*Benzopyrene,* a component of coal tars (not itself a mutagen but may be metabolically activated by enzymes), causes tumors in some animals. Intermediate product shown to be a potent mutagen.	I. B. Weinstein

TABLE 2 *History of Radiation Carcinogenesis*

Year	Radiation	Investigator
1895	*X rays* discovered.	W. Röentgen
1902	*X rays* induce skin cancer.	Frieben
1907	*Ultraviolet light* induces skin cancer in human.	W. Dubreuth
1930	*X rays* cause cancer in mice.	C. Krebs
1944	*X ray–induced leukemia* in radiologists.	H. March
1945	*Atomic bomb explosions* in Hiroshima and Nagasaki cause leukemia and some other forms of cancer.	

TABLE 3   *History of Hormonal Carcinogenesis*

Year	Hormone	Investigator
1928	Breast cancer induced in castrated male mice by grafting mouse ovaries under their skin.	W. Murray
1932	Breast cancer induced in male mice by injecting them with extracts of mouse ovaries.	A. Lacassagne
1938	Breast cancer induced in male mice by injecting them with diethylstilbestrol, a synthetic female sex hormone.	A. Lacassagne
1945	Breast cancer resulted from the combined action of hormones, the mammary tumor virus, and genetic background.	National Cancer Institute scientists
1971	Vaginal cancer in adolescent girls caused by the ingestion of diethylstilbestrol by their mothers during pregnancy.	A. Herbst

TABLE 4   *DNA Viruses Associated with Cancer in Humans*

Year	Virus	Disease
1964	Epstein-Barr virus (EBV)	Burkitt's lymphoma Nasopharyngeal cancer
1967	Hepatitis B virus	Liver cancer
1977	Papilloma viruses	Cervical cancer

TABLE 5   *History of Hereditary Carcinogenesis*

Year	Scientific Advances	Investigator
1866	Principles of heredity defined as the sum of qualities and potentialities transmitted from ancestor to descendant.	G. Mendel
1902	It is proposed that abnormal chromosomes lead to cancer.	T. Boveri
1933	A strain of mice (Ak) is developed with high incidence of leukemia.	J. Fruth
1935	A strain of mice (C3H) is developed with high incidence of breast cancer.	L. Strong
1935	A strain of mice (C58) is developed with high incidence of leukemia.	E. G. MacDowell
1971	A hypothesis is proposed that leads to the discovery of one family of cancer genes, tumor-suppressor genes.	A. Knudsen
1976	Discovery of the first member of a second family of cancer genes called oncogenes.	M. Bishop and H. Varmus
1987	Discovery of a gene that suppresses the metastatic potential of cancer cells.	P. Steeg

TABLE 6   *Cancers Caused by Environmental Factors*

Agent	Site of Cancer
Sunlight	Exposed skin (rodent ulcer, squamous carcinoma, melanoma)
Use of "kangri"[a] and "dhoti"[b]	Skin of abdomen and thigh
Chewing betel, tobacco, snuff	Mouth
Reverse smoking (passive inhalation of cigarette smoke)	Palate
Smoking	Mouth, pharynx, larynx, bronchus, esophagus, bladder
Alcoholic drinks	Mouth, pharynx, larynx, esophagus
Aflatoxin	Liver
Schistosomiasis	Bladder, liver, large intestine
Atomic bomb radiation	Leukemia, most other forms of cancer
Polychlorinated biphenyls (contaminated cooking oils)	Liver

[a]Kangri is a container to hold hot coals
[b]Dhoti is a diaper-like garment
SOURCE: Adapted from table by Sir Richard Doll, introduction to vol. 1 of *Origin of Human Cancer*, ed. H. H. Hiatt, J. D. Watson, and J. A. Wisten (Cold Spring Harbor, N.Y.: Cold Spring Harbor Laboratory Press, 1977).

TABLE 7 *Cancers Caused by Occupational Exposure*

Agent	Occupation	Site of Cancer
Ionizing radiations, radon	certain underground miners (uranium, fluorspar, hematite)	Bronchus
X rays, radium	radiologists, radiographers, luminous dial painters	Skin, bone
Ultraviolet light	farmers, sailors	Skin
Polycyclic hydrocarbons in soot, ore	chimney sweeps, manufacturers of coal gas, many other groups of exposed industrial workers	Scrotum, skin
2-Naphthylamine, 1-naphthylamine	chemical workers, rubber workers, manufacturers of coal gas	Urinary bladder
Benzidine, 4-aminobiphenyl	chemical workers	Urinary bladder
Asbestos	asbestos workers, shipyard and insulation workers, brake liners, cigarette-filter makers	Bronchus, lung, pleura, and peritoneum
Arsenic	sheep-dip manufacturers, gold miners, some vineyard workers, ore smelters	Skin, bronchus
Bis (chloromethyl) ether	makers of ion-exchange resins	Bronchus
Benzene	shoemakers, workers with glue, varnishes, etc.	Bone marrow (leukemia)
Mustard gas	poison-gas makers	Bronchus, larynx paranasal sinuses
Vinyl chloride	polyvinyl chloride manufacturers	Liver
Chrome ores	chromate manufacturers	Bronchus
Nickel ore	nickel refiners	Bronchus, nasal sinuses

TABLE 7 *continued*

Agent	Occupation	Site of Cancer
Isopropyl oil	isopropylene manufacturers, hardwood furniture makers, leather workers	Nasal sinuses

Source: Adapted from table by Sir Richard Doll, introduction to vol. 1 of *Origin of Human Cancer*, ed. H. H. Hiatt, J. D. Watson, and J. A. Wisten (Cold Spring Harbor, N.Y.: Cold Spring Harbor Laboratory Press, 1977).

TABLE 8   *Cancers Caused by Medical Procedures or Prescribed Drugs*

Agent	Site of Cancer
Diagnostic or therapeutic X rays	All sites
Thorium	Bone
Thorotrast	Liver, spleen
Radium RA^{224} injected	Bone
Polycyclic hydrocarbons	
in coal tar ointments	Skin
in liquid paraffin	Stomach, colon, rectum
Alkylating agents melphalan, cyclophosphamide	Leukemia
Estrogens	Uterus, breast
diethylstilbestrol (DES)	Vagina, transplacental cervix
Steroid contraceptives	Liver
Androgens	Liver
Arsenic	Skin, lung
Chlornaphazine	Urinary bladder
Phenacetin	Kidney
Immunosuppressive drugs	Brain, lymphatic system, other sites
Hemodialysis	Kidney

Source: Adapted from table by Sir Richard Doll, introduction to vol. 1 of *Origin of Human Cancer*, ed. H. H. Hiatt, J. D. Watson, and J. A. Wisten (Cold Spring Harbor, N.Y.: Cold Spring Harbor Laboratory Press, 1977).

TABLE 9 *Human Oncogenes Isolated from Cancers*

Oncogenes	Chromosome Location	Site of Cancer
c-*hst*	unknown	Stomach
c-*mas*	6	Breast
c-*met*	7	Bone
c-L-*myc*	1	Lung
c-N-*myc*	2	Nerve
c-N-*ras*	unknown	Various
c-*trk*	1	Colon

TABLE 10 *Human Leukemias and Lymphomas Exhibiting Specific Chromosome Translocations Involving Oncogenes, Immunoglobulin Genes, and T-cell Receptor Genes*

Disease	Chromosome Translocations	Activated Oncogenes	Mechanism of Activation
Burkitt's lymphoma	8 and 2, 14, or 22	c-*myc* on chromosome 8	c-*myc* activated by enhancers of immunoglobulin genes on chromosomes 2, 14, and 22
Chronic lymphocytic leukemia	11 and 14	*bcl*-1 on chromosome 11	*bcl*-1 gene activated by enhancer of immunoglobulin gene on chromosome 14
Follicular lymphoma	14 and 18	*bcl*-2 on chromosome 18	*bcl*-2 gene activated by enhancer of immunoglobulin gene on chromosome 14
T-cell leukemia	8 and 14	c-*myc* on chromosome 8	c-*myc* activated by enhancer of T-cell receptor of gene on chromosome 14

TABLE 11   *Human Cancers with Amplified Protooncogenes*[a]

Cancer	Protooncogenes
Carcinoma of lung, colon, breast, and cervix	c-*myc*
Myelocytic leukemia	
Carcinoma of lung	L-*myc*
Small-cell carcinoma of lung; neuroblastoma	N-*myc*
Adenocarcinoma of the breast, ovary, and stomach	c-*erb*-B-2 (neu, HER-2)
Squamous-cell carcinoma, astrocytoma (brain)	c-*erb*-B-1
Carcinoma of stomach	K-*sam*

[a]When detected, gene amplification varies in most cancers from twentyfold (L-*myc* in carcinoma of the lung) to seven hundredfold (N-*myc* in neuroblastoma).

TABLE 12   *Oncogenes in the Diagnostic Laboratory*

Cancer	Oncogene Alteration	Usefulness
Adenocarcinoma of lung	Point mutation of K-*ras*	Prognosis
Carcinoma of breast	Overexpression of *erb*B	Prognosis
	Amplification of *erb*B	Prognosis
	Amplification of *myc*	Prognosis
Neuroblastoma	Amplification of N-*myc*	Prognosis and selection of therapy
Acute lymphocytic leukemia	Fusion of oncogenes *bcr/abl*	Accurate diagnosis; distinguish from other leukemias; appropriate selection of treatment
Chronic myelogenous leukemia	Translocation of *bcr/abl*	Diagnosis

SOURCE: Adapted from table in M. J. Bishop, "Molecular Themes in Oncogenesis," *Cell* 64 (1991).

TABLE 13 *Human Cancers Associated with Loss of Function of Tumor-Suppressor Genes on Specific Chromosomes*

Childhood Cancers	Chromosomal Location[a]	Tumor-Suppressor Gene[b]
Retinoblastoma, osteosarcoma	13	Rb1
Wilms tumor	11	WT1
Rhabdomyosarcoma, hepatoblastoma	11	Not named
Neuroblastoma	1	Not named
Adult Cancers		
Breast, cervix, bladder, lung, prostate	13	Rb
Breast, lung, colon, brain, others	17	p53
Familial colon cancer	5	APC
Colon	18	DCC
Neurofibromatosis type 1	17	NF1
Familial kidney cancer	3	Not named
Acoustic neuromas	22	Not named
Small-cell carcinoma of lung	3	Not named
Multiple endocrine neoplasia of parathyroid, pancreas, pituitary, and adrenal gland	11	MEN-1
Liver	16	Not named

[a] Although the specific chromosomal locations of some of these representative tumor-suppressor genes are known, others have not been mapped with accuracy.

[b] Molecular clones of Rb, p53, WT1, DCC, and NF1 have been obtained.

TABLE 14 *Alterations of Oncogenes and Tumor-Suppressor Genes in Specific Human Cancers*

	Affected Genes	
Cancers	Oncogene	Tumor-Suppressor (Chromosomal Location)[a]
Breast	erbB (*neu*, HER) myc	p53 (17) Rb (13) (3) (11)
Colon	K-*ras*	p53 (17) APC (5) DCC (18)
Lung	myc L-*myc* N-*myc* raf	p53 (17) Rb (13) (3)
Brain (astrocytomas, acoustic neuromas)	erbB (*neu*) myc N-*myc* ras sis	p53 (17) (22)
Neuroblastoma	N-*myc* N-*ras*	(1)

[a]Chromosomal locations of tumor-suppressor genes on chromosomes 1, 3, and 11 have not been named or accurately mapped.

GLOSSARY

Adduct The product resulting from the combination of two compounds (*add*ition prod*uct*).

Allele One of several alternative forms of a gene occupying a given position on a chromosome.

Amino Acid Sequence The linear order of the amino acids in a peptide or protein.

Amplification To increase in number, for instance, the copies of oncogenes in certain cancer cells.

Angiogenic Factors Proteins that increase the number of blood vessels in a tissue.

Antigen Any object that, upon injection into a vertebrate, is capable of stimulating the production of antibodies.

B Lymphocytes Small lymphocytes that synthesize and secrete humoral antibodies upon antigenic stimulation.

Carcinogen An agent that induces cancer.

Cell The fundamental unit of life; the smallest body capable of independent reproduction. A cell is always surrounded by a membrane.

Cell Culture The *in vitro* growth of cells isolated from multicellular organisms.

Cell Differentiation The process whereby descendants of a common parental cell achieve and maintain specialization of structure and function.

Cell Fusion Formation of a single hybrid cell with nuclei and cytoplasm from different cells.

Central Dogma The basic relationship among DNA, RNA, and proteins: DNA serves as a template for both its own duplication and the synthesis of RNA; RNA, in turn, is the template in protein synthesis.

Chemical Carcinogen Any chemical substance capable of causing cancer.

Chromosomes A discrete unit of the total genetic information carrying many genes. Each chromosome consists of a very long molecule of double-stranded DNA.

Clone   A group of cells all descended from a single common ancestor.

Codon   A sequence of three adjacent nucleotides that codes for an amino acid (or chain termination).

Colony   A group of contiguous cells, usually derived from a single ancestor, growing on a solid surface.

Complementary Chain of DNA   A strand of DNA that matches another strand by virtue of having the appropriate base at each position to pair with the base on the other strand (guanine with cytosine and thymine with adenine). This is the essential concept of Watson and Crick's double-stranded model of DNA.

Deletions   Loss of a section of genetic material from a chromosome. The size of the deleted material can vary from a single nucleotide to sections containing a number of genes.

Deoxyribonucleotide   A compound that consists of a purine or pyrimidine base bonded to the sugar 2-deoxyribose, which in turn is bound to a phosphate group.

DNA (Deoxyribonucleic Acid)   A polymer of deoxyribonucleotides. The genetic material of all cells.

DNA Sequence   The precise order of the four nucleotides—adenine (A), guanine (G), cytosine (C), and thymine (T)—as they are linked together to form the DNA chain. This DNA sequence encodes the genetic information of an organism.

DNA Transfection   The transfer of DNA into cells in culture. The foreign DNA can associate with the host chromosome and be expressed as an identifiable phenotype.

Dominant   An allele that exerts its phenotypic effect when present either in homozygous (two copies) or heterozygous (one copy) form.

Enhancers   DNA elements of varying length that can be located upstream or downstream from a gene and enhance gene transcription.

Enzymes   Protein molecules capable of catalyzing chemical reactions.

Epithelium   The tissue that acts as a covering or lining for any organ or organism.

Established Cell Line   Cultured cells of a single origin, capable of stable growth for many generations.

Estrogen   Female sex hormone produced by the ovary.

Exon   That portion of DNA that codes for the amino acid sequences, that is, expressed DNA sequences.

Fibroblasts   Differentiated cells that grow very well in culture. They have the spindle shape and growth rate of connective tissue cells.

Gene   That portion of DNA at a specific locus that controls the production of a polypeptide or a portion of a protein. A gene can consist of combinations of contiguous exons and introns.

Gene Therapy   Treatment of a disease caused by a defective gene by insertion of a normal gene into the cells.

Gene Transcription Synthesis of an RNA molecule by polymerization of nucleotides complementary to a DNA template. This RNA molecule is a precursor of messenger RNA and represents a faithful complementary copy of the DNA sequence from which it is transcribed.

Genetic Information The information contained in a sequence of nucleotide bases in a DNA (or RNA) molecule.

Genome The total of genetic information contained in a haploid set of chromosomes. Also used to denote the total genetic information contained in a cell or in an organism.

Genotype The genetic constitution of an organism (to be distinguished from its physical appearance, or phenotype).

Growth Factor A type of protein that stimulates cell growth and differentiation.

Hormones Chemical substances (protein, amino acid derivatives, or steroids) synthesized in one organ of body that stimulate functional activity in cells of other tissues and organs.

Inbred Mouse Strains Lines of mice that have been produced by brother-sister mating or other schemes of intrafamilial breeding, usually for more than twenty generations, so that each mouse within that line is genetically identical to every other mouse with a high degree of probability.

Insertional Mutagenesis The process of interrupting the structure of a gene by inserting foreign genetic information.

Intron That portion of DNA that is not expressed in the amino acid sequences. Also known as *intervening sequences.*

Leukemia Form of cancer characterized by extensive proliferation of nonfunctional immature white blood cells (leukocytes).

Linked Genes Genes that are located on the same chromosome and that therefore tend to segregate together.

Locus That portion of a chromosome on which a gene is situated.

Long Terminal Repeat (LTR) A repetitive element of the integrated provirus that is generated during viral DNA synthesis and contains the transcription control elements that regulate virus expression.

Lymphatic Tissues Those tissues, including lymph nodes and vessels, thymus, and spleen, that produce and contain the lymphocytes.

Lymphoma Cancer of lymphatic tissue.

Messenger RNA RNA derived from the exons of DNA that directs the synthesis of a peptide.

Metastasis The spread of cancer to sites distant from the original tumor.

Mitosis Process whereby chromosomes duplicate and segregate, accompanied by cell division.

Mutagens Chemical agents and physical agents, such as radiation or heat, that raise the frequency of mutation greatly above the spontaneous background level.

Mutation An inheritable change in a chromosome.

Oncogene   The gene responsible for inducing the transformed cancer phenotype.

Phenotype   The observable properties of an organism, produced by the genotype in cooperation with the environment.

Polypeptide   A polymer of amino acids linked together by peptide bonds.

Promoter   Region on DNA at which RNA polymerase binds and initiates transcription.

Protease   An enzyme that digests proteins.

Protooncogene   A gene present in normal cells that promotes cells to proliferate and differentiate into specialized cells.

Provirus   The state of a virus in which it is integrated into a host cell chromosome and is thus transmitted from one cell generation to another.

Regulatory Genes   Genes whose primary function is to control the rate of synthesis of the products of other genes.

Resection   The surgical removal of part of a tissue or organ.

Retinoblastoma   A cancer of the eye that occurs in infants and children under the age of five.

Retrovirus   Small RNA virus consisting of virally coded glycoprotein in a lipid membrane derived from host cell membranes and an RNA-nucleoprotein core. The small genome of these viruses contains a gene coding for reverse transcriptase, virion proteins, and often an oncogene.

Reverse Transcriptase   An enzyme that directs the production of a DNA copy of RNA (the reverse of transcription).

Sarcoma   Cancer of connective tissue.

Stroma   The material in which cells are embedded.

Transcription   Production of an RNA copy of DNA, as in the production of messenger RNA.

Transfection   The genetic modification induced by the incorporation into a cell of DNA purified from cells or viruses.

Translation   The process whereby the genetic information present in a messenger RNA molecule directs the order of the specific amino acids during protein synthesis.

Translocation   The movement of a segment of a chromosome to a new site on another chromosome.

Tumor   Mass formed by the uncontrolled proliferation of cancerous cells.

Tumor-Suppressor Gene   A gene present in normal cells that constrains the proliferation of normal cells and of cancer cells.

Tumor Virus   A virus that induces the formation of a tumor.

Viruses   Infectious disease-causing agents, smaller than bacteria, which always require intact host cells for replication and which contain either DNA or RNA as their genetic component.

Wild-type Gene   The form of a gene (allele) commonly found in nature.

Wilms' Tumor   A kidney cancer that occurs in infants and young children.

BIBLIOGRAPHY

AARONSON, S. A. 1991. "Growth Factors and Cancer." *Science* 254: 1146–52.

ALLISON, M. 1992. "Mammography Trial Comes Under Fire." *Science* 256: 1128–30.

AMES, B. N. 1983. "Dietary Carcinogens and Anticarcinogens." *Science* 221: 1256–64.

ANDERSON, W. F. 1992. "Human Gene Therapy." *Science* 256: 808–13.

BEARDSLEY, T. 1994. "A War Not Won." *Scientific American* 270: 130–38.

BENEDICT, W. F., A. L. MURPHREE, A. BANERJEE, ET AL. 1983. "Patient with 13 Chromosome Deletion: Evidence That the Retinoblastoma Gene Is a Recessive Cancer Gene." *Science* 219: 973–75.

BISHOP, M. J. 1982. "Oncogenes." *Scientific American* 246: 82–90.

———. 1991. "Molecular Themes in Oncogenesis." *Cell* 64: 235–49.

BOVERI, T. 1914. *The Origin of Malignant Tumors.* Jena, Germany: Gustave Fischer Verlag.

BRODEUR, G., R. C. SEEGER, M. SCHWAB, H. E. VARMUS, AND M. J. BISHOP. 1984. "Amplification of N-*myc* in Untreated Human Neuroblastomas Correlates with Advanced Disease Stage." *Science* 224: 1121–24.

BURKITT, D. 1991. "Are Our Commonest Diseases Preventable?" *The Pharos* 54:19–21.

CAIRNS, J. 1978. *Cancer, Science and Society.* San Francisco: Freeman.

CARNEY, D. W., AND K. SIKORA, eds. 1990. *Genes and Cancer.* New York: Wiley.

CATALONA, W. J., D. S. SMITH, T. L. RATLIFF, ET AL. 1991. "Measurement of Prostate-specific Antigen in Serum as a Screening Test for Prostate Cancer." *New England Journal of Medicine* 324: 1156–61.

CHLEBOWSKI, R. T., ET AL. 1991. "Adjuvant Dietary Fat Intake Reduction in Postmenopausal Breast Cancer Patient Management." *Breast Cancer Research and Treatment* 20: 73–84.

CHODAK, G. W., R. A. THISTED, G. S. GERBER, ET AL. 1994. "Results of Conservative Management of Clinically Localized Prostate Cancer." *New England Journal of Medicine* 330: 242–48.

CLEARY, M. L. 1993. "A Promiscuous Oncogene in Acute Leukemia." *New England Journal of Medicine* 329: 958–59.

CLINE, M. J. 1994. "Mechanisms of Disease: The Molecular Basis of Leukemia." *New England Journal of Medicine* 330: 328–36.

COHEN, J. 1993. "Cancer Vaccines Get a Shot in the Arm." *Science* 262: 841–43.

COMINGS, D. E. 1973. "A General Theory of Carcinogenesis." *Proceedings of the National Academy of Science, USA* 70: 3324–28.

Committee on Diet and Health, Food and Nutrition Board, Commission on Life Sciences, National Research Council. 1988. *Diet and Health: Implications for Reducing Chronic Disease Risk.* Washington, D.C.: National Academy Press.

COOPER, G. M. 1990. *Oncogenes.* Boston: Jones and Bartlett.

CULOTTA, E., AND D. E. KOSHLAND, JR. 1993. "p53 Sweeps Through Cancer Research." *Science* 262: 1958–61.

DARNELL, J., H. LODISH, AND D. BALTIMORE. 1986. *Molecular Cell Biology.* New York: Scientific American Books.

DAVIDSON, N. E. 1992. "Tamoxifen—Panacea or Pandora's Box?" *New England Journal of Medicine* 326: 885–86.

DEVITA, V. T., JR., S. HELLMAN, AND S. A. ROSENBERG, eds. 1989. *Cancer, Principles and Practices,* 3rd ed. Philadelphia: Lippincott.

DOLL, R. 1978. "An Epidemiological Perspective of the Biology of Cancer." *Cancer Research* 38: 3573–83.

DULBECCO, R. 1987. *The Design of Life.* New Haven and London: Yale University Press.

EBBELL, B., trans. 1937. *The Papyrus Ebers. The Greatest Egyptian Medical Document.* Copenhagen: Levin and Munksgaard.

ELVERSON, T. C. 1964. "Spontaneous Regression of Cancer." *Annals of the New York Academy of Science* 114: 721–35.

FEARON, E. R., AND B. VOGELSTEIN. 1990. "A Genetic Model for Colorectal Tumorigenesis." *Cell* 61: 759–67.

FIDLER, I. J. 1990. "Critical Factors in the Biology of Human Cancer Metastasis: Special Lecture." *Cancer Research* 50: 6130–38.

GARDNER, M. B., S. RASHEED, R. W. SHIMIZU, ET AL. 1977. "Search for RNA Tumor Virus in Humans." In *Origins of Human Cancer,* ed. H. H. Hiatt, J. D. Watson, and J. A. Wisten, pp. 1235–52. Cold Spring Harbor, N.Y.: Cold Spring Harbor Laboratory Press.

GATOFF, E. 1982. "Cancer Genes and Development: The Drosophila Case." *Advances in Cancer Research* 37: 33–67.

GREENSPAN, E. 1991. Quoted in *Los Angeles Times.* November 13.

GROSS, L. 1983. *Oncogenic Viruses,* 3rd ed. Oxford: Pergamon Press.

HARRIS, C. C. 1993. "p53: At the Crossroads of Molecular Carcinogenesis and Risk Assessment." *Science* 262: 1980–81.

HARRIS, C. C., AND M. HOLLSTEIN, 1993. "Clinical Implications of the p53 Tumor-Suppressor Gene." *New England Journal of Medicine* 329: 1318–25.

HARRIS, J. R., M. E. LIPPMAN, V. VERONESI, AND W. WILLETT. 1992. "Medical Progress: Breast Cancer." (Three parts.) *New England Journal of Medicine* 327: 319–28, 390–98, 473–80.

HEALY, B. 1993. "Mammograms—Your Breasts, Your Choice." *Wall Street Journal* December 28.

HEBER, D. 1984. "Diet, Nutrition and Cancer." *UCLA Cancer Bulletin* 11: 5–8.

HENDERSON, B. E., R. K. ROSS, AND M. C. PIKE. 1991. "Toward the Primary Prevention of Cancer." *Science* 254: 1131–38.

———. 1993. "Hormonal Chemoprevention of Cancer in Women." *Science* 259: 633–38.

HIATT, H. H., J. D. WATSON, AND J. A. WISTEN, eds. 1977. *Origin of Human Cancer.* Cold Spring Harbor, N.Y.: Cold Spring Harbor Laboratory Press.

HOFFMAN, M. 1992. "New Clue Found to Oncogene's Role in Breast Cancer." *Science* 256: 1129.

HUEBNER, R. J., AND G. J. TODERO. 1969. "Oncogenes of RNA Tumor Viruses as Determinants of Cancer." *Proceedings of the National Academy of Sciences* 64: 1087–93.

KLURFELD, D. M., AND D. KRITCHEVSKY. 1986. "Update on Dietary Fat and Cancer." *Proceedings of the Society for Experimental Biological Medicine* 183: 287–92.

KNUDSON, A. G. 1971. "Mutation and Cancer: Statistical Study of Retinoblastoma." *Proceedings of the National Academy of Sciences* 68: 820–23.

———. 1985. "Hereditary Cancer, Oncogenes and Antioncogenes." *Cancer Research* 45: 1437–43.

———. 1993. "Antioncogenes and Human Cancer." *Proceedings of the National Academy of Sciences* 90: 10914–21.

LEVINE, A. J. 1992. "The p53 Tumor-Suppressor Gene." *New England Journal of Medicine* 326: 1350–51.

LEVINE, A. J., J. MOMAND, AND C. A. FINLAY. 1991. "The p53 Tumor-Suppressor Gene." *Nature* 351: 453–56.

LI, F. P., J. F. FRAUMENI, JR., J. J. MULVIHILL, W. A. BLATTNER, M. DREYFUS, M. A. TUCKER, AND R. W. MILLER. 1988. "A Cancer Family Syndrome in Twenty-four Kindreds." *Cancer Research* 48: 5358–62.

LIOTTA, L. A. 1992. "Cancer Cell Invasion and Metastasis." *Scientific American* 266: 54–63.

LIOTTA, L. A., P. S. STEEG, AND W. G. STETLER-STEVENSON. 1991. "Cancer Metastasis and Angiogenesis. An Imbalance of Positive and Negative Regulation." *Cell* 64: 327–37.

McClintock, B. 1950. "Multiple Loci in Maize." *Carnegie Institute, Washington Year Book* 49: 157–67.

Makita, M., G. Sakamoto, et al. 1990. "Natural History of Breast Cancer Among Japanese and Caucasian Females." *Gan To Kagaku Ryoho* 17: 1239–43.

Marshall, C. J. 1991. "Tumor-Suppressor Genes." *Cell* 64: 313–26.

Marshall, Eliot. 1991. "Breast Cancer: Stalemate in the War on Cancer." *Science* 254: 1719–20.

Marx, J. 1991. "Zeroing In on Individual Cancer Risk." *Science* 253: 612–16.

———. 1993. "Learning How to Suppress Cancer." *Science* 261: 1385–87.

———. 1993. "How p53 Suppresses Cell Growth." *Science* 262: 1644–45.

———. 1993. "Gene Defect Identified in Common Hereditary Colon Cancer." *Science* 262: 1645.

Miller, A. D. 1992. "Human Gene Therapy Comes of Age." *Nature* 357: 455–60.

Morra, M., and E. Potts. 1987. *Choices, Realistic Alternatives in Cancer Treatment*, 1st rev. ed. New York: Avon Books.

Morrison, A. S., C. R. Lowe, B. MacMahon, et al. 1976. "Some International Differences in Treatment and Survival in Breast Cancer." *International Journal of Cancer* 18: 269–73.

Murphree, A. L., and W. F. Benedict. 1984. "Retinoblastoma: Clues to Human Oncogenes." *Science* 203: 1028–33.

Norman, C., T. P. Gately, and D. De Francesco. 1993. "Breast Cancer Research: A Special Report." *Science* 259: 616–32.

Oesterberg, J. E., S. K. Martin, E. J. Bergstralk, and F. C. Lowe. 1993. "The Use of Prostate-Specific Antigen in Staging Patients with Newly Diagnosed Prostate Cancer." *Journal of the American Medical Association* 269: 57–60.

Park, M., and G. F. Vande Woude. 1977. "Principles of Cell Biology of Cancer: Oncogenes." In *Cancer, Principles and Practice*, ed. V. T. DeVita, Jr., S. Hellman, and S. A. Rosenberg. Philadelphia: Lippincott.

Poiesz, B. J., F. W. Ruscetti, A. F. Gadzar, P. A. Bunn, J. D. Minna, and R. C. Gallo. 1980. "Detection and Isolation of Type C Retrovirus Particles from Fresh and Cultured Lymphocytes of a Patient with Cutaneous T-cell Lymphoma." *Proceedings of the National Academy of Sciences* 77: 7415–19.

Powell, S. M., et al. 1992. "APC Mutations Occur Early During Colorectal Tumorigenesis." *Nature* 359: 235–37.

Powell, S. M., G. M. Petersen, A. J. Krush, et al. 1993. "Molecular Diagnosis of Familial Adenomatous Polyposis." *New England Journal of Medicine* 329: 1982–87.

Reddy Premkumar, E., R. K. Reynolds, E. Santos, and B. Mariano. 1982. "A Point Mutation Is Responsible for the Acquisition of Transforming

Properties by the T24 Human Bladder Carcinoma Oncogene." *Nature* 300: 149–52.

ROBERTS, L. 1993. "Zeroing in on a Breast Cancer Susceptibility Gene." *Science* 259: 622–25.

ROSENBERG, S. A., P. AEBERSOLD, K. CORNETTA, ET AL. 1990. "Gene Transfer into Humans—Immunotherapy of Patients with Advanced Melanoma Using Tumor-Infiltrating Lymphocytes Modified by Retroviral Gene Transduction." *New England Journal of Medicine* 323: 570–78.

ROUS, P. 1911. "Transmission of a Malignant New Growth by Means of a Cell-Free Filtrate." *Journal of the American Medical Association* 56: 198.

SAGER, R. 1986. "Genetic Suppression of Tumor Formation: A New Frontier in Cancer Research." *Cancer Research* 46: 1573–80.

SANDROFF, R. January 1992. "Gallup Poll: Cancer #1 Personal Health Concern." *Oncology Times* 18.

SHIMIZU, S., W. J. SCHULL, AND H. KATO. 1990. "Cancer Risk Among Atomic Bomb Survivors." *Journal of the American Medical Association* 264: 601–4.

SHIMKIN, M. B. 1977. "Contrary to Nature." *U.S. Department of Health, Education, and Welfare Publication No. (NIH) 76–720.*

SIDRANSKY, D., ET AL. 1992. "Identification of *ras* Oncogene Mutations in the Stool of Patients with Curable Colorectal Tumors." *Science* 256: 102–5.

SOLOMON, E., J. BARROW, AND A. D. GODDARD. 1991. "Chromosome Aberrations and Cancer." *Science* 254: 1153–60.

STANBRIDGE, E. J., AND P. C. NOWELL. 1990. "Origins of Human Cancer Revisited: Meeting Review." *Cell* 63: 867–74.

TANNOCK, I. F., AND M. BOYER. 1990. "When Is Cancer Treatment Worthwhile?" *New England Journal of Medicine* 323: 989–90.

TORECHETTE, N. 1990. "Tumor Suppressors: A New Arena in the War Against Cancer." *Journal of NIH Research* 2: 62–66.

VOGELSTEIN, B., AND K. W. KINZLER. 1992. "Carcinogens Leave Fingerprints." *Nature* 355: 209–21.

WATSON, J. D. 1987. *Molecular Biology of the Gene*, 4th ed. Menlo Park, Calif.: W. A. Benjamin.

WEINBERG, R. A. 1989a. "Oncogenes, Antioncogenes and the Molecular Basis of Multistep Carcinogenesis." *Cancer Research* 49: 3712–21.

———. 1989b. *Oncogenes and the Molecular Origins of Cancer.* Cold Spring Harbor, N.Y.: Cold Spring Harbor Laboratory Press.

———. 1991. "Tumor-Suppressor Genes." *Science* 254: 1138–45.

WEISSMAN, B. E., P. J. SAXON, S. R. PASQUALE, ET AL. 1987. "Introduction of a Normal Human Chromosome 11 into a Wilms' Tumor Cell Line Controls Its Tumorigenic Expression." *Science* 236: 175–80.

ZUR HAUSEN, H. 1991. "Viruses in Human Cancer." *Science* 254: 1167–72.

INDEX